Dal Shh
8-21-07

Tewksbury Tales Press, LLC.
9 Patriot Hill Drive
Basking Ridge, NJ 07920

First Tewksbury edition 2007
Original published in the United States by arrangement with the author.

Book and cover designed by David Stark
Set in Adobe Garamond Pro
Cover illustration by Michael Morgenstern
Manufactured in the United States of America

Library of Congress Control Number: 2007900940
ISBN-13: 978-1-934160-00-8

Silence of the Bunnies

of the

TALES OF LIFE, LOVE AND SURVIVAL

DAN STARK

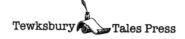
Tewksbury Tales Press

TABLE OF CONTENTS

ABOUT THE AUTHOR

Dan Stark was born in Oxnard, California, in 1952. The first fifty years of his life were uneventful. He grew up in Orlando, Florida, in the time before Disneyworld and during the height of the Cold War. This, and frequent encounters with the large roaches common in Florida, may have contributed to his decision to study first philosophy and then law. He practiced law for twenty-seven years, the last twenty-one at AT&T, before retiring as a Vice President of the company in August 2004. This is his first book.

Dan has been married twice, and currently lives in New Jersey with his daughter's dog Coop, a very tolerant animal. They live close to where his wife Mary and their daughter Lily live. Dan has a son Hank who graduated with an English degree from the University of Michigan and will be attending law school at Northwestern this fall. He also has a stepson Zane who he hopes to be able to brag about at some future point.

Dan has Parkinson's disease, but that cannot alone explain the contents of this book. He is too damn happy given his problems. He shares the secrets to remaining happy while your life goes into the toilet in this book. You would expect to pay hundreds of dollars and have to go to therapy for years to learn such skills, but Dan has priced the book, including these secrets, very reasonably. Dan is that kind of guy.

DEDICATION & ACKNOWLEDGEMENTS

For my mother, who passed away November 10, 2004, and to Mary, Henry and Lily, without whose presence in my life this would have been a very different book.

Those of you who don't like this book may blame Bob Victor and his mother-in-law Mary Edsall; Craig Stoltz, health editor at the Washington Post; my developmental editor Laurie Rosin; my brother David Stark; and friends and unpaid literary advisers Peter Morgan and Vicki Fleiss. Without their help and encouragement, you would not be holding it in your hands.

Finally, I want to thank Margaret Tuchman, whose courage and grace battling Parkinson's disease has made me realize how light a burden illness can become when you spend your time, as she does, helping others rather than worrying about yourself.

Introduction:

How I Wrote This Book and Proved That God Exists

This book is a celebration of life, despite increasing evidence of my own mortality. I do not say that to start off on a sad note. To the contrary, I accept that we all must die at some point, although if death comes for me too early I intend to put on a pair of Groucho glasses and pretend to be someone else.

I had always been healthy, almost abnormally so. I had never been in the hospital except to visit someone else, and a health crisis to me was my annual cold. Then, about ten years ago, when I was in my early forties, things began to deteriorate—quickly. I started things off with a torn ligament in my knee, followed in rapid succession by a diagnosis of Parkinson's disease, open heart surgery, brain surgery, and to bring us current, or heck, just for the fun of it, hand surgery last month resulting from my attempt to put ice cream into a ceramic bowl.

I have managed to stay without new crises for three weeks now so what, you may ask, am I whining about?

I have no complaints. Ignore for the moment the knee and hand surgery. These were annoying rather than dangerous and therefore did nothing to shape my outlook on life.

The heart and brain surgery, on the other hand, made me realize that I was playing chess with Death for keeps. I had fended him off this time with what I believe is a new variation to the Queen's Gambit Declined opening. After feeling his breathing on my neck—an unprofessional tactic he used to distract me during the game—I could not return to life as a corporate lawyer as if nothing had happened.

I became a night owl because the Parkinson's symptoms included muscle cramps in my back that made it difficult to sleep more than a couple hours at a stretch. There is not much you can do at three in the morning without waking others who don't want to be woken, so I began to write. I discovered miraculously that writing, about the only thing I could do, was the thing I most wanted to do.

In the year that followed, I wrote about two dozen stories/essays. After two of them appeared in the Washington Post, I thought that they might be good enough to publish as a book. I put them together and sent the lot to an editor who had worked on numerous successful books. I had the usual fantasies of new writers that she would call me soon after she started to read, unable to contain her wonder that words could be so elegantly employed, or the human condition so poignantly explained. Not this time. She tried with great tact to tell me that there were problems with my manuscript.

Collections of essays don't sell unless written by God, and even then do less well than His other works. Worse, my essays mixed fact and fancy, confusing everyone from publishers to book stores as to whether this was fiction or non-fiction. Worst of all, I made fun of just about everybody—insurance companies and their employees, Republicans, political science majors, creationists, evolutionists, evangelists, Islamic extremists, accordion players, most men and all women. If those I criticized were, in addition to all their other faults, petty enough not to buy the book for this reason, then I was in trouble. "You are in trouble," the editor advised.

I had a small number of books printed, and took them to one of those mega-department stores near where I lived. The store had miles of shelf space where you could find things like The Three Stooges on VHS. I showed the store manager the book. He thumbed through it and then tossed it unceremoniously back to me, saying "Not interested." When I asked him why, he responded, "Didn't you see our slogan when you entered the store? Like I said, not interested." I hadn't looked up to read their slogan. I did now. It read, "We sell everything except mixed genre literature."

I looked back at the man and saw him putting some sheet music that had fallen on the floor back on the shelf. It was a transcription of a Mahler symphony for the accordion. I backed away in horror and nearly tripped over a political science major restacking items on the bottom shelf as I ran from the store.

What could I do? I had poured my heart into this book. I called God. As usual there was no answer. I said in a louder voice, "God, if you're there, please pick up the phone. I really need to talk to you." His voice response system kicked in. I heard His voice say: "This is God. Please listen to this entire message as my menu has changed recently. If you are a first time caller and are calling for forgiveness of a grievous but not mortal sin, dial one."

This was not my first time calling, and I knew that listening to the entire menu could take years. I hung up and went to look for Him instead. I found Him muttering, trying to fill in a rebate coupon for His cell phone. He saw me, stood up laughing, and told me that He was enjoying reading my writing more than He had expected. While I tried to figure out whether that was a compliment, He gave me a hug, fracturing two of my ribs. God didn't know His own strength.

Without much coaxing, I began to tell Him of my woes. "I've heard much worse," He said. "Get over it." Then He asked how, given its many flaws, I expected to sell more than one or two copies to close relatives. I told Him that because all the essays/stories contained autobiographical material, I had changed a few things here and there, and then used my skills in metaphysics to turn the manuscript into a "Memoir." But I also told Him that I was hoping that He could make the book part of a few million people's life scripts.

"Life what…?" He asked. I told Him about a recent book that described how He planned people's lives. He laughed, and then became annoyed. "I guess I could, although there are billions of you. Do you have any idea how exhausting that would be?" He snorted and resumed, "You know, humans are very aggravating. You think I have nothing better to do than to solve your problems. Just yesterday, some Islamic fellow who had detonated a bomb strapped to his waist asked me to put him back together so that he could become intimate with the virgins he had met here. You'd think that being God would earn me some respect. Instead, Clarence Thomas gets the interesting and important cases to decide, and I'm expected to reassemble private parts from a million pieces exploded all over the place. I feel some rain coming on; I hope you know how to swim."

I let Him calm down, which He always did. Well, almost always. He grinned, and promised to finish reading my book, saying that—assuming He liked it—He would speak to Oprah to see what could be done. Gradually at first, and then picking up speed, it began to sell. It's good to have God (and Oprah) on your side.

For those of you who don't believe in Him, or doubt what I have been saying, can you offer any other explanation of how you are holding my book in your hands, despite all its obvious shortcomings? It's a miracle is what it is, and there is only one source of those.

This book is broken into Parts, a more expansive concept than chapters. The Parts make occasional progress in telling you about my life, but they also are home to the sideways pursuit of thoughts on assorted matters which I pursue to a greater extent than would be justified if this were a mere memoir. I call such detours "interludes" to let you know not to expect too much autobiographical forward progress while reading them.

I also have chosen to start with my triumph over Parkinson's disease. No, I haven't beaten the disease physically. Unless a cure is found, it ultimately will beat me. My triumph is one of spirit, because I refuse to accept it as an excuse to mope. I start with the account of my fight against the disease, even though it means starting with the present and then circling back to cover my youth, in the hope that reading about it will make you less critical of any mistakes or offensive remarks you may find within these pages. Were I to delay telling of my struggle with this dreaded disease until the end of the book, you might instead extend such tolerance to the author of the book you read next. What would be the point of that?

PART I:

PARKINSON'S DISEASE AND ALL THAT JAZZ

I have known I had Parkinson's disease for nearly a decade. Early in 1997, I noticed that my fifth finger on my right hand would twitch while I was shaving. It hadn't twitched for the first forty-five years of my life, so I figured it wasn't supposed to. I went to a neurologist who told me that I did *not* have Parkinson's disease, but rather essential tremor, an annoying but comparatively harmless condition. It was just as well I didn't celebrate too much, because his diagnosis was wrong.

My symptoms worsened slowly but noticeably during the year. I made an appointment with a neurologist who specialized in brain disorders for New Years Eve, the first appointment I could get. He confirmed what I strongly suspected by that point—I had Parkinson's disease. I still didn't know much about the disease, but I remember telling my wife (and believing it myself) that the disease was so slow moving that "they" were almost certain to find a cure well before it became a real issue for me.

I also remember thinking that it was important that the world not know that I had the disease. I don't know why I reached that conclusion, but I think it is a fairly common reaction. I wanted to be me, not someone with Parkinson's. I threw myself into my work harder than ever, partly to keep from thinking about my illness, and partly to prove that even the healthiest of my peers couldn't keep up with my new pace.

In other words, I did just about everything wrong for the first few years.

First Interlude:
Living Large with Parkinson's [1]

When I was diagnosed with Parkinson's disease, I had little knowledge of what lay ahead. Most people share that ignorance. Though the reactions of the few I told about my condition were typically intense, with exclamations of great pity or sorrow, this was often followed by a very honest "What exactly is Parkinson's?"

This proved harder to answer than you'd think. Doctors seemed reluctant to say much. I was told that everyone's experience was different. It seemed a manageable disease, at least to me, at least then.

For six years after my diagnosis, I maintained my frenetic lifestyle, which mixed big-corporation lawyering with a typically busy family life. I didn't think about it much because, frankly, I didn't have the time.

Then came a rapid acceleration of symptoms. I was unprepared for the ferocity of the assault. For six years, I had ingested an increasingly abundant cornucopia of pharmaceutical industry produce. Now, the length of the relief I could squeeze from a dose dropped from about four hours to less than one and a half.

When drugs were not effective my speech became soft and stilted, and my back became the pain epicenter of my world, my muscles contracting into a large knot. The pain became intense if I stayed in

---

[1] This Interlude appeared initially, with minor differences, in the *Washington Post*, June 21, 2005

bed more than an hour or two, making sleep something that other people did.

In order to keep going and present a picture of health by day, I started taking more and more medication without my doctor's knowledge. This did not go well. I suffered periods of uncontrollable shaking. My hands became numb.

Within two weeks, I slid from a place where my symptoms were largely under control to one where they were spinning out of it. I was sleep-deprived, in severe pain, and shifting between flopping like a flounder and experiencing the near immobility of a stump.

As I tried to adjust to my new reality, the realization hit me that the progressive nature of the disease meant that in six months what I was experiencing now would seem like "the good old days." The thought hit me like a hard punch to the stomach. I actually sucked in my breath and sat down.

I could almost feel my will draining away. I began to think about suicide, not because I was depressed, but because it seemed like a rational response to my situation. I picked out a particularly solid looking tree at the bottom of a long hill near my house that I knew I could drive into at a very high speed. That would be my way out if things got too much to bear. I mention this not to stretch for melodrama or appeal for sympathy, but because it is true.

I hid behind a screen of e-mail banter with friends. Only my wife, Mary, was on the inside, and we were each living in our own worlds.

I had no right to expect help from her. We had each retreated into our own fortresses some time ago, and she had been dealing with her own problems with little help from me. But on the day I hit bottom, she emerged from her fortress and rescued me. Looking much prettier than John Wayne but every bit as heroic, she put everything else aside, put her arms around me, and told me that she loved me.

This time it was the disease that was caught off guard. It thought it had me down. Mary gave me the strength to fight back. Since then I have found new things that have helped. While not yet ready to declare victory, I am definitely unwilling to accept defeat. Sadly, I could not prevent Mary from retreating to the safety of her fortress afterwards. She had helped me when I needed it, but I was back on my own.

Why am I sharing these very private experiences? After I was diagnosed, it seemed that people didn't want to tell me about what lay ahead for fear of depressing me. Yes, the facts about Parkinson's can be brutal. Remaining blissfully ignorant until your world collapses, however, strips you of the ability to plan ahead and defend yourself.

Following is my attempt to sketch a road map for those diagnosed with this lousy disease. I don't pretend to cover the medical part, for which you will receive copious advice, some of it useful and some of it correct. This is about how to think about your life.

Parkinson's disease is caused by the premature death of the brain cells that create a chemical called dopamine. Dopamine is an enabler that helps the brain transmit instructions to the muscles. Without it, actions that require muscular participation—moving, eating and breathing, to name just three—can get dicey.

To get an idea of Parkinson's effect on the body, imagine what happens when you try to use a motor that has run out of oil. Being an idiot with mechanical things long before I had Parkinson's, I did that once to a Sears' lawnmower. Everything trembled, there were terrible noises, and finally it just locked up, billowing smoke. It has occurred to me in moments of severe sleep deprivation that my disease is somehow linked, in spirit if not in cause, to my mistreatment of that mechanical companion.

Naming this disease after an English physician with a kind-sounding name does nothing to help people understand it. The name doesn't convey suffering; it sounds like you can't remember where you left the car at the mall.

Getting public support to fund research requires something that sounds more fearful. My proposal is "Spreading Muscle Death." It not only captures what is going on in a very melodramatic way, it carries a hint of contagion. Though Parkinson's of course does not spread from person to person, I am confident that a name that sounds like it might, would produce a nice up-tick in contributions to find a cure.

People need to know you have Parkinson's before it really becomes apparent. This will prepare them for the difficult times ahead. It will also provide access to one of the few benefits that come with this disease: a license to enjoy life.

Anybody with a pulse deserves time to stop and smell the roses, of course. Most people don't get it. The undiagnosed do not find it easy to slow down. They're healthy and they are expected to act like it. They rush from thing to thing, because that is how we try to balance the modern pulls of family, job, the search for happiness, etc.

We Parkinson's types can slow things down to a speed where they can be savored without fear of criticism, especially once our movements start to become more labored. In the time it takes our fingers to pull the petals from a flower to determine if we are loved, we have the opportunity to embellish and extend the range of the emotions involved ("She loves me. Well, I thought so originally but lately I just don't know. She loves me not. She's changed and this is never going to work.") In time, we are able to add poetry and even short stories to the process, so slow do our fingers become. There is richness to the fabric of life that we are able to notice and enjoy that the undiagnosed cannot imagine.

Early Parkinson's symptoms are usually minor: a little stiffness, a few twitches, and a vague psychic unrest that weakens inhibitions. In exchange for these relatively mild burdens, one gets immediate sympathy from those who think you're already immobile and choking on food. These things will happen in the future. For now, enjoy the best of both worlds: sympathy and kind treatment without severe bodily degradation. To get the breathing space, however, you must let people know that you have the disease. Nothing disclosed, nothing gained.

If you don't take advantage of this, you are wasting a perfectly good disease. Don't get depressed that you are sick. Look around you. Everyone you see is also dying, maybe slowly, maybe not. Because they don't realize this, they are willing to extend you kindness while expecting none themselves. We live in a game show culture where those who first identify what is killing them get showered with sympathy and benefits, while those who don't discover their cause of death until much later get no rewards for their mortality. It doesn't really matter who actually dies first. Be the first to know you're dying and win!

The truth is that those who do not learn of their demise until they are close to it frequently get very little time to enjoy life. Parkinson's, if diagnosed early, presents a rare opportunity. The disease is horrible enough to command immediate sympathy, but progresses slowly enough to leave you substantial time to enjoy the good without experiencing too much of the bad. Don't waste the opportunity moping about it, or you will miss the good and be left with only what you're spending your time moping about.

Accept your good fortune modestly, but accept it. There are roses that need smelling. The opportunity falls to you.

One key "but" here: Disclosing early is important, but that doesn't mean complaining all the time.

Yours is not the worst situation that one can imagine. There are many diseases that trump Parkinson's in their misery index that are the "no feet" response to your "no shoes" situation. Childhood leukemia, inoperable brain cancer, quadriplegia, and massive third-degree burns . . . the list is long.

So share the news and get on with it. No one likes to be around someone constantly bemoaning his or her fate. Don't worry, you'll get good treatment without needing to look like your dog died. It worked for me. Of course, my dog did die . . . . Actually, both dogs. And a cat. And two bunnies, my mother, my mother-in-law and. . . . But all of that's another story.

See? You didn't want to hear about all that. Nobody does.

Wouldn't life be great if we were freed from all the little fears that constrain our behavior? Have you ever wanted to speak your mind at work but were held back for fear that it would damage your career? Now you can do so without fear of long-term consequences, because frankly, the long term just isn't among your problems right now.

The same is true socially. If you see a woman and are struck by her charm (assuming you are single), ask her out. Some will say no because of your condition, and some would have said no if your health were impeccable. But you know better than anyone that it is not social rejection that will kill you. So take some risks!

More important, the "you" that emerges once the myriad petty fears are stripped away will be so impressive that she might even say yes. In fact, this may be the "you" you should have been all along.

The buoyancy that results from dropping one's fears about what others think is absolutely startling. The knowledge that time is short, coupled with a willingness to take risks, unleashes an energy that makes even the need for sleep seem a pity.

So put this aside. Go have the time of your life, to the extent your symptoms permit it. Proceed without fear. Pursue your passions and whims. You will know when it is time to resume reading. And who knows? By then we may have a cure for Spreading Muscle Death.

PHASE TWO

I hope you had a long and colorful interlude. I assume if you're reading this that we still do not have a cure and you're starting to hurt. Let's look at what lies ahead.

At some point the symptoms start worsening. Your life becomes a function of the pills you take. The king is Sinamet, the giver of synthetic dopamine, which lets our muscles respond almost as if we were normal. It can provide relief for many years.

But, as you are now discovering, your own dopamine-producing cells are continuing to dive off a cliff. The result is that you need to take more Sinamet to keep the symptoms at bay.

Without the drug, you become almost immobile. Your body becomes wooden, you develop roots that hold you to the ground, and squirrels begin to look at you with interest.

On the other hand, take too much medicine for too long and you begin experiencing those uncontrollable movements that make people with Parkinson's unwelcome at exhibits of artisan glass.

Threading the needle between stopped and flopped inevitably becomes trickier. Some doctors can do this much better than others and can buy you precious extra years. Don't feel bad about switching doctors. It's your life, not theirs.

The best guide to what lies ahead, alas, is the questionnaire routinely used to score the progression of the disease.

Can you dress yourself?

Do you drool excessively, only at night or during the day?

Do your feet stick to the floor when you try to walk?

Can you turn over in bed?

Have you fallen, or experienced any hallucinations or dementia?

Have you choked on your food?

Call me slow on the uptake, but it eventually dawned on me that they asked these questions because someday I would experience most of these. In a way, it is a gentle way to reveal the unpleasant future.

In contrast to your experience in the first phase, you are now paying a serious price for any sympathy you earn. The rose-smelling can be very difficult and infrequent. But the disease still can be managed if you are careful.

The advice, then, is clear: Find a good doctor to minimize the symptoms and continue enjoying what you can. Don't worry about Phase 3; there will be time enough when it arrives.

PHASE THREE

What do you do when your symptoms become too severe for the ordinary arsenal of treatments to handle?

There are plenty of things to try: clinical trials with experimental drugs, brain surgery to implant pulsating electrodes, intensive exercise routines, etc. All have their adherents, and all can give some relief to some people. I am investigating them all. But none works well enough to protect you permanently from the continuing onslaught. So here are your instructions:

Keep your sense of humor and don't lose hope. Fight this thing as long as you can, and then fight it some more. Maintaining hope as the disease advances will become hard to do. It is no fun being a stump. Or a flopping fish.

During those times when the drugs have not worked well, I've experienced what it feels like to be on the inside of a body that the brain cannot move. It is not blinding agony, but it is so persistent a mental and physical ache that I cannot imagine living with it for a long time. But would you want to give up if the cure were only days or weeks away?

How long will it take before a cure is available? To help understand the answer, I have drawn on my corporate background and constructed a project management timeline. (Project management timelines, I learned, do little to make success more likely, but they do make you look better explaining your failures.)

By assigning reasonable time periods to raise funds, identify promising areas of medical research, engage in protracted fights with opponents of stem cell research, perform the research, negotiate with drug companies, negotiate with the FDA, perform clinical trials, again and again, and then file papers seeking approval, and wait, I have determined that a cure could be made available in—bear with me here while I do the calculations . . . forty-six years.

Wait, I almost forgot: Winnie the Bush (our president of Little Brain) was reelected. He finds it politically expedient to accommodate the noisy, increasingly theocratic right wing of his party by blocking critical research that would use stem cells. (See, now that I'm sick I'm saying all the things I used to hold back. I am livin' large!) Add four years to account for his second term and the lingering damage he is likely to do, and you have an even fifty years.

Fifty years is too long for most of us to wait. I'll be dead by then anyway. Hopefully, we will have future presidents with bigger brains or hearts than the incumbent.

Other countries are not constraining their stem cell research. Japanese companies are in the game, adding their technical prowess to the hunt. That ought to save a decade, easy. Great Britain's in on the chase, too; knock off another five years.

Money is time; with more funding, we can shave more years from the tally. Who knows how much sooner we can make it happen? Recall that contributions to your favorite Parkinson's foundation are tax-deductible in this life, and may improve your accommodations in the next. (Or you may come back as a goat; your guess is as good as mine.)

Eventually we will beat this. Those with the disease can then rejoin the mainstream and die of something else, ideally much later. Death may be our common destination, but there are different roads one can take there.

There's a road I know of that would allow me enough time to walk a bit further with my kids, discussing law with my son and watching my little girl, her eyes dancing with mischief, as she picks dandelions and dodges my efforts to prevent her blowing their seeds on our lawn. It's the first turn on the left, just past a cure for Parkinson's. I'd like to take it.

First, I have a task to tend to. I am finishing watching the sunrise in St. Thomas (yes, the St. Thomas in the U.S. Virgin Islands). It looks like another beautiful day, so it may be difficult to squeeze in even a modest dose of self-pity before brunch. In fact, I may not even try. If it rains tomorrow, I can try to make it up.

☆ ☆ ☆

It took more than Parkinson's disease to wake me up. I did try to take better care of myself, and made a point of actually going for annual physicals.

That's how they picked up the fact that my heart had enlarged and that I needed heart surgery to repair a leaky valve. The heart surgery, much more than the Parkinson's symptoms, forced me to look at my life. It had an immediacy that a slow moving disease lacked. It also forced me to take some time off from work and gave me the opportunity to think deep thoughts during the six week convalescence when I could do little else.

My life, which seemed a success when I didn't think much about it, didn't fare nearly as well when I did. My closer look made me realize I was at risk of leaving this planet having done almost everything I was supposed to do, and very little of what I wanted to do.

I began trying to "seize the day." I ordered a Porsche, a symbolic act that was largely ineffective, but did allow me to drive a really nice car. I loved the car, but there were a number of problems in my life that a Porsche couldn't fix. I listed on a piece of paper the things going awry, as well as a shorter list of the things giving me joy. I stared at the lists, not knowing what to do with them, until I remembered that I had forgotten to include on the first list the deaths of the rabbits that my wife had given our daughter.

For whatever reason, writing about our two rabbits brought my emotions to the surface, and cauterized my feelings that "life" was treating me unfairly. Writing it changed me. The notion of taking my own life if the symptoms got too bad had empowered me previously, giving me the ability to think about my condition without fear. After I wrote the story, that exit seemed out of the question. I would never give up or give in to the disease. It might and likely would kill me, but it was going to be one hell of a fight.

SECOND INTERLUDE:
SILENCE OF THE BUNNIES [2]

A few years back, God's warranty on my health expired.

Understand that I had never been in the hospital, never missed a day of work, and had just completed my first "century"—a 100-mile bike ride. So it seemed unfair that I tore a ligament in my knee playing tennis and required an operation.

Okay, you say, grin and bear it. I agree. But then that little twitching in my pinky on my right hand got annoying, so off I limped to the doctor. Parkinson's disease. Damn.

---

[2] This Interlude appeared initially, with minor differences, in the *Washington Post*, Oct. 19, 2004

Time to watch my health more closely, get annual physicals and so forth. Going to my physical resulted in a chest X-ray showing an enlarged heart. No big deal—this was not something that required immediate attention. I had up to four months to fix a problem valve.

Now I know that lots of people have medical problems. Pets do as well. Within the last year, our cat and both dogs died. They were old.

So was my mother-in-law. She lived with us because of health problems brought on by diabetes. She died in our home shortly after the second of the dogs, but not before she would pass out in various rooms, falling heavily to the floor and breaking various parts of her body in each fall, and sometimes coloring the floor with her blood.

I'm not drawing a comparison between human and animal deaths, but I'm clustering the deaths here because they acted strongly on my seven-year-old daughter who loved both grandmother and dogs without reserve.

These things happen. Of course, it's a bit of a strange coincidence that on the day of my mother-in-law's funeral, my own mother had a stroke, and was no longer able to stand on her own. Perhaps she was worried about my father, who passed out in an airport in France and cracked his head open. His pacemaker has helped some, but it seems his heart is failing. That makes it difficult for him to help her.

I'm not really complaining. I run an efficient mental zoo, and I am able to put all these worrisome beasts in their cages for the evening where they cannot disturb me. Then I drink a glass of wine and relax, allowing the worries of the day to deal with themselves for a while. I do that privately now, because my wife has her own problems to deal with, including health challenges no less daunting than mine. We seem to go our own ways more and more.

There are wonderful things in my life, too. My daughter gives me all the emotional love I can handle. My son makes me proud every time I look at him: a six foot two inch hunk who graduated from the University of Michigan, can dunk a basketball or turn the girls' heads depending on his mood, and who exudes a warmth and humanity that are visible just by looking at him. He also has rejected all fatherly advice and is going to go to law school. I couldn't be more proud.

He's going to be awfully embarrassed when he reads this.

The war between good and bad in my life would have left me without a sense of direction but for the emotional guidance provided from an unexpected source.

We had moved into a lovely house out in the country, but our luck seemed to go bad about the time we moved in. Our animals fared no better. I started wondering whether we were intruding where we shouldn't, for instance whether we were living above an Indian burial ground. Before I became paranoid about the place, we brought into our lives two bunnies, Horton and Boinger, who lived in a charming rabbit hutch in our backyard.

In the early days they added to my daughter's delight—they were brothers, one brown and one black. Except for a few times when they acted differently than I thought brothers should act, they were an uplifting joy to feed, hold, or engage in games they seemed prepared to repeat endlessly.

Sadly, during a particularly violent thunderstorm, the hutch blew over and the bunnies were freed. We couldn't catch them despite repeated efforts to do so. As a result, they lived in our backyard having the best of both worlds: freedom from confinement and a free lunch.

Freedom does not come without risk, and after about two weeks, Boinger stopped making appearances. To an adult, he was missing and presumed dead. To my daughter, that was just one of the possibilities. More likely, he had met up with savvy rabbits that persuaded him to come live in their place while he learned the tricks of survival in the wild.

No such fantasy was possible with Horton. One evening I heard a plaintive, half-wailing, half-agonizing shriek outside, but close to our house. It was, I came to realize, the sound a rabbit makes when being turned into a meal.

Horton was almost certainly in the jaws of another animal that had already done some damage, but was carrying off its victim for a final attack followed by a gruesome but very natural dinner.

The wailing was repeated over the course of the next several minutes, lasting perhaps twenty seconds a wail, with an increasing length of time between each outburst. It started close to the house and moved gradually deeper into the woods. Dusk had come, and without knowing what I would do, I went outside with a flashlight to look for the source.

I never saw the fox, which is what I believe it was, but the light caused a reflection of two eyes, which receded along with the wails moving away from me.

Then the wailing stopped, and I knew in my heart that Horton was gone. As horrible as the wailing was, the silence that followed was devastating.

We never saw Horton again. I hadn't particularly loved the bunnies while we had them. But I missed them now, and I was haunted by the sound that Horton had made. In my mind, it wasn't solely an expression of physical pain, although there was plenty of that. It also was the lament of a living creature knowing its life was about to end, expressing an instinctual desire to live despite the terrible circumstances in which it found itself.

The silence of that night has stayed with me. It reminds me of the tremendous thirst for life we animals share. As I think about my desire to see myself and those I love end their stay on this planet with grace and dignity, I can't help but wonder whether we will want to continue suffering in the jaws of disease rather than letting go. I had always intended to live well until I no longer could do so, and then end my life with dignity. The bunny's lament makes me wonder whether I have it in me to give up the fight. If Horton wanted to live this badly, despite living a lonely existence, intensely frightening to a creature prepared only for the dangers of a pet store, there had to be something here that I had missed.

My mother is very ill now, and living in a way that she once said she would never want. As my Parkinson's advances I will eventually face the same predicament. I don't think I will be able to face death with less passion than Horton. I am going to thrash around, fight the fox and scream to the heavens about it. Despite everything going on in my life, I cannot allow myself to be carried away without resistance in the jaws of my attacker, and quietly devoured. You may get me, fox, but not without a fight.

Attitude will carry you far, but at some point you need both will and a few new weapons. The disease was making my current weapons ineffective, and I decided to take the last clear step to clear the symptoms from my daily life. I chose to get brain surgery, which—despite the claims of its adherents—is still a risky procedure. For me it was painful as well, though it needn't be in the hands of a skilled and caring surgeon. But as I sit here nine months after surgery, and look at it now, it was clearly worth it, and yes, I would do it again but with a different surgeon.

THIRD INTERLUDE:
WIRED FOR HOPE [3]

I am by nature impulsive. I was in the Virgin Islands on vacation with my daughter when I decided to have brain surgery. Being in such a heavenly place made me both optimistic about what life could be and intolerant of how Parkinson's disease was slowly eliminating my ability to enjoy it.

When I returned home, I called my neurologist and told her I wanted to have deep brain stimulation, or DBS.

DBS involves the implantation of electrodes into very specific areas of the brain. When connected to a power unit and to controllers implanted in the chest, the electrodes deliver signals that interfere with the Parkinson's-induced signals from the brain, reducing or at least temporarily eliminating the quaking, quivering, rigidity and slowness that characterize the disease. The device can be set in so many permutations that it takes weeks or months to program it correctly. Set the voltages too high, and your hands or feet feel electrified; too low, and you need to supplement them with more medication. "Just right" feels pretty damn good.

The benefit of the procedure lies in its ability to intervene electrically rather than chemically. As Parkinson's advances, the medication one needs increases to the point where the patient faces an unwelcome

---

[3] This Interlude appeared initially, with minor differences, in the *Washington Post*, June 27, 2006

choice: either take enough and deal with the shaking and gyrating movements the medication causes, or reduce the dosage and allow the Parkinson's symptoms, which can be similar to those side effects of the drugs, to take over your body. As time passes, your body veers between being difficult to move and moving uncontrollably, with less and less time in the comfort zone between.

DBS changes the dynamic. It does not totally replace medication, but it greatly reduces the need for it. In my case, at its best, DBS has allowed me to function while taking only about a quarter of my previous medication. That enabled me to reduce the chemicals in my blood, permitting me to avoid my transformation into a stump without triggering bouts of shaking. As life with Parkinson's goes, this is not so bad.

One must remember though, that *DBS does nothing to deal with the underlying disease, and is therefore a temporary reprieve from Parkinson's symptoms, and not a cure.* It is, however, a reprieve without the horrific side effects that the current drug therapies generally cause.

Prior to the surgery, the level of drugs in my blood would build up during the day so that by evening I would nearly writhe out of my chair. That was bad at home; in public, it was a disaster. My courage was wilting under the stares of strangers and, worse, the sympathetic looks of horror from friends. Like many others with advanced Parkinson's, I was at risk of transforming my home into a prison, a place I could leave but seldom if ever did.

DBS changed all that, though not overnight and not easily. My surgery was excruciatingly painful. It is true that there are no nerve endings in the brain, as the maker of DBS implants likes to tell prospective users. One has to reach the brain first, however, and that means drilling through the skull.

There is about a 1-in-20 chance of things going very wrong during the surgery. I didn't worry. I did not believe my luck would be so bad as to draw the single short straw among 19 long ones. What did preoccupy my thoughts before surgery was the prospect of staying awake during the entire four- to six-hour procedure.

DBS is done in two stages, generally spaced five to seven days apart. On the first day of surgery, they implant the electrodes in the brain. On the second, they insert the battery and control units in your chest, and the wires just beneath the skin, connecting the stuff in your brain to the stuff in your chest. Generally, you are in the hospital only one night, after the first day of surgery.

On the day of my first surgery, I was told to arrive at the hospital at four in the morning. I did so, and spent most of the next seven hours getting checked in (total elapsed time: six minutes) and waiting (six hours fifty four minutes). Perhaps it was to soothe restless patients that they had the woman I privately named "Bright and Perky" handling the admissions process in Same Day Surgery. She too arrived at four in the morning, but unlike me and the majority of other patients, she arrived fully functional and incredibly cheerful even at that ungodly hour. There was just no sag in the woman, either physically, or in her indefatigable good spirits.

Seeing someone like that in the otherwise dark and drab world of same-day surgery was unnatural and unexpected, yet there she was calling my name, checking me into the hospital and putting a plastic bracelet around my wrist that identified me by name and birth-date, so that they would know that I was there for brain surgery and not to have a leg amputated.

A mere hour or two later, when they called me to go through a door and enter the world of pre-operative care, I not only went voluntarily, I even feigned a nonchalance as I walked past her that I thought would impress her with my courage. For all I know, she might have been impressed, despite her equally brave pretense to have forgotten all about me. It was hard to tell with her, especially since she didn't look up as I walked by.

Once in the world of pre-operative care, thoughts of beauty were soon left behind. I was asked to put on two hospital gowns, one facing in each direction, apparently a new technique used to overcome the gown's inherently indiscrete design. But because I had been instructed not to take my Parkinson's medications the day of surgery, I was shaky and got so tangled that I emerged from a dressing room in disarray and unintentionally put on a show. That's okay; worse things were to come.

When my neurosurgeon arrived, things started to happen. He had wanted an MRI of my brain, but that had not been done. And apparently there was a shortage that day of the people who move patients from place to place. The surgeon was impatient, and the next thing I knew, the director of the MRI facility, a likable young man who told me to call him "MRI Mark," was wheeling me to the MRI room, explaining as he misjudged a turn and clipped a wall hard that this was not something he normally did.

Before the MRI could be taken, a metal cage called a halo needed to be attached to my head. It looked like a prop from a bad science-fiction movie. The halo is used to immobilize the head and to assist in the location of the precise targets for the drill. As the neurosurgeon twisted the first of four screws into my head to secure the halo, I grimaced. The local anesthetic was not yet effective. I let him know this, and he promised to give me more painkiller "in a minute," just as soon as he finished what he was doing.

As he moved on to the second screw, I remember thinking that giving me more painkiller after he finished was a little like closing the barn door after killing all the animals inside. He screwed the remaining screws in halfway, and then went back to each screw and screwed it in until it was tight.

I was dazed and thought the pain was a necessary rite of passage, a sort of Parkinson's hazing ritual. It was only later that I learned from other brain surgery veterans that the pain was entirely avoidable. One simply needed to wait briefly for the anesthetic to take effect.

I began thinking of the neurosurgeon as "Dr. Evil." I recognize this may be unfair to him. I doubt he's really evil. More like indifferent to patient pain. But "Dr. Indifference" just sounds weird.

Being conscious during surgery reveals a whole different realm of experience. I was able to overhear arguments between my neurologist and Dr. E. on the critical issue of electrode placement. I was able to hear one of the physician's assistants adding numbers to determine drilling coordinates and making error after error—each of which the surgeon fortunately caught and corrected. While waiting to go into the OR, I observed another medical team wake a patient from anesthesia just enough to hold a pen and sign a consent form. I overheard an anesthesiologist, unhappy to learn that a patient was allergic to a particular drug, call the pharmacy, listen to the possible adverse reactions, and respond, "Well, let's just try it and see how it goes."

Despite the unnecessary pain I experienced, this surgery changed my life. True, there have been plenty of annoying back-and-forths with my neurologist to tweak the settings. But the sweet spot that lies between too much juice and too little is sweet indeed.

Just knowing I have a device in my head that can control Parkinson's symptoms has given me hope and patience. I have found myself thinking about having fun again. My mood has started to lighten.

More people need to know about this surgery. Despite its flaws, it is better than any alternatives I've encountered, and I've exhausted all approved medications and have participated in two clinical trials of new drugs.

My endorsement of DBS is not unqualified. There are some things the surgery makes better (movement); others it makes worse (balance and speech). For most patients, the things it makes better are more significant than those it makes worse, but anyone considering it should be aware of all the consequences.

Finally, the implanted apparatus itself could be improved. It runs on batteries that need to be replaced every few years, and the power units are large enough to be plainly visible if you are not wearing a shirt. I want the good people at Medtronic, the maker of the device, to know that I am not being critical. But I've had plenty of time to think, and there seem to be some pretty obvious improvements that could be made.

For instance, Rolex makes watches that generate electricity from body movements. Why not apply that to a DBS unit? I figure one good episode of dyskinesia could keep my unit going for a month. That would be a huge improvement over their present product, which requires surgery to change the batteries every few years.

Or take the iPod Nano, which packs a lot more features into a much smaller package than the unit in my chest. Maybe Medtronic should simply license the technology. And not just for the size advantage: The DBS wiring under the skin goes from the chest and wraps around the ear on its way to the brain. Perfect! Implant the iPod's headphone cord at the same time, and just drop it off at the ear. Figure out how to turn it off and on, and make selections, and we could listen to music on demand within our own heads!

Of course, there is also wireless technology. If my home computer network can produce a signal strong enough for some hacker at the curb to steal my Social Security number, why can't a DBS unit toss a signal from my clavicle to my brain? Or allow me to communicate with others who have similar gear inside their bodies to allow a very private conversation, brain to brain?

If the scientists at Medtronic learn to think outside the head, they may come up with something so nifty that even those without Parkinson's will want it.

For now, I am content with what I have. The pain of getting it implanted is fading from memory, and while I still have more tinkering with the settings ahead of me, even today I have less symptoms and take less medication than before.

I figure one can either worry about the future or enjoy what the present has to offer. I confess I sometimes allow worries to get the better of me. Trying to have fun with the things we must deal with is so much more satisfying that I invariably return to this approach.

It's not because I'm brave. It's because I am alive, damn it, and that is a whole lot more than you can say about people who are not. After all, who would have guessed five years ago that I would have brain surgery and a few weeks later buy a tennis racket? But I did.

I just hope the 10-year layoff has helped my game.

The most difficult part about writing about the future is that it has not yet happened. We live in a universe where things either happen at random or in patterns too complex to grasp without drinking way too much. As a result, predicting what may happen in the future is a very tough business.

There are exceptions of course. My future experience with Parkinson's disease appears to be one of those. It is predictable what happens when the disease is left to run its course. Without dopamine, the chemical your dead brain cells used to make, muscles in your body continue to become less and less responsive. Swallowing becomes a constant challenge, breathing becomes difficult, and sleeping becomes impossible. It's not a pretty way to wrap up one's life.

This is my future; it is the present for many others. They too had hopes and dreams that the disease would be cured by now. Yet while each day brings death and misery to an increasing number, we move only fitfully towards a cure.

If I am honest, and assess the speed with which the disease is taking over my body and compare that to the progress being made towards a cure, I must accept that this is my future too. I have good friends who have had the disease longer than I; they have even less chance to escape. Yes, I have had brain surgery which has alleviated the symptoms for now. But it does nothing to stop the disease, and at some point in the future the benefits of the surgery will be engulfed by the disease's onward march.

I would scream if that would do any good. It does not. I have tried and can report based on my own empirical observations that railing against having the disease does not cure it. Neither does wishing it would go away, fantasizing that the next bite of my peanut butter and jelly sandwich would miraculously cure me, or trying to pretend I never had it in the first place. I know, because I have tried all these too.

The disease *is* curable. It is a riddle like any other that requires applying human ingenuity, resources and time to solve. The problem is that we are applying very few resources to this particular riddle, making it fairly easy to predict that absent some stroke of very good, and unearned, luck, the cure will come too late for me and most of the people I know.

I read recently that legislation funding the various middle-eastern wars we are engaged in has been signed into law, providing another ninety billion dollars or so towards our efforts to kill people who do not like us in Iraq and Afghanistan. I don't profess to know enough to know whether spending all that money, not to mention the lives of our soldiers, has been for a good, or a mistaken, cause.

Whatever the answer, it is nonetheless disheartening to be one of more than a million Americans facing a future ruined by Parkinson's, knowing that with a billion dollars committed by the government to research we could probably find a cure. That is a huge amount of money. There are a number of other diseases that make many other millions miserable or dead; a billion dollars each would produce cures for a number of them.

It isn't even a close call: there is something far more compelling about spending our money to kill people who do not like us in foreign countries than to save the lives of Americans here at home.

No doubt you have already concluded that I am a bleeding heart liberal willing to throw dollars at every do-gooder cause that comes along. For that reason, I have come up with a fiscally responsible alternative to the funding legislation that just passed. In rough form, it would be as follows:

First, take ten billion of the ninety and spend a billion dollars per disease for ten different diseases. The goal, a reasonable one, would be to find cures for half of them. To aid in passage, I can promise that I would provide learned scientists who would testify that with this kind of funding, we actually have a wonderful chance of finding cures for a number of them, helping millions of Americans. Consider it a short-term investment: the amount of money the country would realize in increased productivity, all taxable of course, and reduced medical expenses to address the symptoms of disease (much of which is paid for today by the government) would offset the initial expense in a very brief period.

Second, to broaden our coalition, take another ten billion dollars and give it to auto companies, energy companies and others to do research on energy alternatives to make us less dependent on middle-eastern oil. Take another five billion dollars to spend on anything and everything in the districts of key members of Congress. Yet another five billion dollars goes to Halliburton without competitive bids for them to do whatever they want so long as it will make the Vice President happy.

Third, there are some people in foreign countries who don't like us and may well be better off dead. I really don't know first hand that there are, but I am willing to accept this since we seem to be trying so hard to kill them. So let's cough up thirty billion dollars to do this, a third of what the current plan is. The good news is that while we may not be able to kill as many with thirty as with ninety billion dollars, it seems that the more we spend trying to kill people in foreign countries, the more new enemies we create. In fact we appear to be making more people hate us for every person who already hates us that we are able to kill. Bottom line: My proposal will kill fewer of our enemies but also will make far less new ones, producing a net reduction in enemies as compared to the current plan.

Finally, to prove that I am fiscally conservative, I propose that the last thirty billion dollars be given back to our Treasury, keeping spending down and reducing pressure on interest rates.

You see how this disease causes me to think irrationally? How could I expect the government, which today spends very little, all things considered, on finding cures for this or most other diseases, to spend ten billion dollars to save my and other people's lives? Where could they possibly come up with the money, and why spend it on such nonsense?

Today, the private efforts of a number of different organizations raise tens of millions of dollars a year in search of a cure. It's wonderful, but it is not enough for many of us. Time is life, and we are running out of it. Please forgive me for my effort to rethink the use of that ninety billion dollars. It must be needed or we wouldn't be spending it, right? What if we took just one or two months off from killing the people in foreign countries who don't like us? We could then do all the good things I proposed, and return a few months later and kill them then.

You now see why I don't understand politics. It is so confusing for me to understand what makes some things priorities worth huge expenditures and other things not important enough to spend anything. Thank goodness there are people who understand this so that we don't waste our money on the wrong things.

PART II:

How I Grew Up in Orlando, Florida, and Learned That God Was on Our Side, Especially If You Were White, and That the Only Good Communist Was a Dead Communist

I was born in 1952 in Oxnard, California, a satellite of Los Angeles. I have no clue what part of the ox the "nard" is, but even the best part seemed pretty second-rate compared to being born in the neighboring, beautiful and sunny city of angels. It wasn't easy living on the wrong side of the highway, and this unearned adversity made me realize that I faced an uphill struggle to make my voice heard over the oxen around me. Sometimes we are shaped more by accident than by design.

My father had been crisscrossing the country in search of work. My sister, the eldest, was born on the West Coast; my brother, who came next, was born on the East Coast; and I was born back on the West Coast. I had six months of warm weather and blondes before we moved back East. I don't remember a damn thing about the first six months of my life, so other than reporting that I lived through it, there is nothing more to say.

We moved back to Baltimore, Maryland, and lived there for four years. My father was then working for an aerospace company, Martin Marietta, now Lockheed Martin. The company decided to move a number of engineers and their families to the sleepy southern town of Orlando, Florida, because land was so cheap that they could pay for the move and still come out ahead. I remember very little about life in Maryland. I remember my brother, two years older and to me a full-grown God, picking up a snake thinking it was something else and having it slither out of his hand! He screamed and we then both ran home in tears. I was ready to move.

Today we think of Disney when we think of Orlando. In the late fifties and early sixties it was still a fairly typical southern town. My memories are not the genteel views used in romanticized histories of Southern living. Southern society was rigidly segregated and intolerant, and most of my memories that survive include those elements.

I remember being in a department store in downtown Orlando when I was four or five years old. I was thirsty, and my brother and I were standing in a line to get a drink from a water fountain in the store. There was another water fountain right next to the one for which we were waiting. There was no one in line. I looked at the fountain again to see if anything was wrong. It looked fine, so I went up and drank from it.

My brother, whose two years' age advantage bestowed upon him the ability to read, looked around nervously before pulling me away. He asked me if I hadn't seen the sign. I reminded him that I didn't know how to read. Once outside he told me that the sign had read "colored only," a complement to the "whites only" sign over the fountain for which we had been waiting. I tried to discern whether the "colored only" water had caused any damage, but I couldn't find any. I remember wondering why, if the water was the same, they placed two fountains right next to each other when one would have worked just as well.

We were Jewish. The slaughter of most of the Jews in Europe during the Holocaust had ended less than twenty years earlier. My mother wasn't about to hide, or let us hide, the fact that we were Jewish. On each Jewish holiday, we stayed home from school, though I can't remember ever going to temple. The important thing to her was that people knew that we were Jewish, and that we were proud of it!

Jews weren't quite as bad as blacks in the opinions of most whites, but they were pretty bad for white people. Everyone knew that Jews were rich and had cheated others to get that way. You had to be careful when dealing with us or we would "Jew" (meaning cheat) you. Use of the word Jew to mean cheat was so common that people were surprised that I took offense; surely I wasn't trying to say that Jews didn't have a thing for money or that we had earned it honestly?

The other thing people knew about Jews was that we had killed Jesus. That made it okay to push us around a bit and to refuse us admission to private places where the federal prohibitions on discrimination did not apply. Many communities were restricted. Golf courses and tennis clubs were the most visible places not permitting Jews to become members, but they were by no means the only ones.

When my father was promoted into the top job in Orlando, he created a problem. Martin then was the largest and most important employer in the area. It was customary that the general manager would sit on a number of local boards, and be an honorary member of various other institutions, many of which didn't accept Jewish people. A few decided to invite him to join anyway; most did not. Even at Martin, where he had won more contracts than any other person, resulting in billions upon billions of dollars of business for the company, he was passed over for both raises and further promotions in favor of people who the chairman "was more comfortable with."

My mother was also a first generation American. Her parents had come to this country from Poland. She had no living relatives left in Europe. Poland, unlike Russia, had surrendered to the Germans, and every member of her mother's family who did not leave Poland before the war was killed. As a Jew who had lost so many relatives simply because they were Jewish, mistreatment of blacks simply because they were black, was intolerable. She was an exception. Most Southern whites truly believed that blacks were inferior and clung to language that put the blacks in their "proper place."

It might surprise you that Orlando was a very religious place, despite the bigotry. Somehow, these good people believed in a version of Christianity that was tolerant of racial and ethnic hatred. It left me very skeptical and unsympathetic towards organized religion. Anything malleable enough not to condemn Southern prejudice could not be worth much.

My hero was federal law as established by the Warren Court and implemented by federal district court judges. Yes, they overruled precedents and made the Constitution a living and breathing document, but the country we are now able to have pride in is the result of their doing so. Brown vs. Board of Education, finding that racial separation was inherently unequal, and Miranda vs. Arizona, preventing the use of confessions obtained by isolation or beatings of those arrested, may be the best known of these decisions, but there were many key decisions that broke the backs of bigotry, abuse of power, and imposition of majority religious beliefs on minorities.

Today, when conservatives preach a rejection of the judicial principles that support those decisions, especially when those statements come from justices as freewheeling with precedent and constitutional interpretation as any on the Warren Court ever were, it brings back uncomfortable images from my youth. Most people my age remember the image of George Wallace vowing to block the entry of black students into state universities in the name of states' rights. Fewer have seen the incredibly disturbing photographs of white men and women, picnic baskets pushed to the side, pausing to have photographs taken beside the lynched bodies of blacks hanging from trees. It is never a good time to have bad judges on our highest court, but we should at least be thankful that those who would not have lifted a finger to stop the abuses and privation of huge portions of our population were still in diapers learning to say "momma," "dada," and "states' rights" when the Warren Court lifted us from the depths.

If you believed in God those days, you had to hate communism because it was atheistic. My high school principal concluded I was a commie around the time my mother sent me to school with a note that read: "Please excuse Daniel from school today so that he can attend an anti-war demonstration." In retaliation, he had me kicked out of honor society for failing to participate in a bake sale, or to reimburse the society for the brownie revenues lost. I suspect that in the long history of that society, I am probably the only student stripped of this academic honor for failure to bake cookies.

What saved me from being turned into a radical was going to college in Boston and meeting students who were. I found them as ridiculous as my high school principal had been. They quickly concluded I was a fascist from the South. I remained in the political center and wondered why each extreme didn't just leave me alone and torment each other.

FOURTH INTERLUDE:

PACKAGING—THE LAST COMMUNIST OFFENSIVE OF THE COLD WAR

Timing is everything. I grew up in Orlando, Florida, in the 1950s and '60s. That was too early for Disney, but just right for the Cold War. Orlando was within easy reach of the missiles the Russians had snuck into Cuba, and we would have been a certain target had there been some "heat" introduced into the conflict. The unusually long runways tourists enjoy when they land today in Orlando are a vestige of McCoy Air Force base, which in those earlier times was home to a large group of B-52 bombers. It wasn't a secret; you could see their distinctive, long wings and high tails from the road.

The business of building fallout shelters in people's yards was hopping! Many people had them and would keep them stocked with food, ready for occupancy. My parents never built a shelter for us. It's not that they didn't love us; my father was the head of a project to build an anti-missile missile defense system for the government. It wouldn't have looked good if the man in charge of the missile program, designed to prevent Russian missiles from hitting us, built a shelter in his yard, which only would have been of use if they did.

One of my good friends had a shelter in his yard, so when we wanted to play "nuclear attack" we just played over there.

We also received special training in elementary school—in case of nuclear attack, we were taught to crawl under our desks and not to look out the windows. This last point was important because the brilliance of a nuclear explosion could damage one's eyesight. It was reassuring to know how to protect yourself if the unthinkable happened, although I sometimes wondered whether the desk tops were really strong enough to protect us if the blast were too close.

Fortunately, our school board found reasons why the Supreme Court decisions that limited prayer in public schools did not apply to us. As a result, I had a fine education filled with prayers and religious instruction over the loudspeakers. With the constant talk of possible nuclear conflict, it was comforting to hear the prayers and to learn that God liked us better. As a requirement of state law, we also took a course called "Americanism versus Communism." The textbooks were written by J. Edgar Hoover. The title I remember was "You Can Trust a Communist...to be a Communist." The man's humor is often overlooked.

Because of my intense Cold War training, I was naturally suspicious about the sudden fall of communism. It happened almost painlessly, without our destroying a single Russian city. People danced in the street and declared the cold war over. This facile collapse by our long time foe may have duped some people, but you have to get up pretty early in the morning to fool someone trained to spot communists by J. Edgar Hoover.

Remember *The Iliad,* Homer's story of the Greek assault on the ancient city of Troy? After years of war, the Greeks realized that they could not breach the city's defenses with a frontal assault. Instead, they pretended to give up and boarded their boats, leaving behind a wooden horse with soldiers hidden inside. The Trojans spent their first day of the new peace drinking too much. A few of the more sober ones tried to tidy things up, and hauled the horse within the city walls before going to bed, so that it would be safe.

Big mistake. The Greek soldiers waited until the Trojans were asleep, and then crept out and opened the gates to the city. The rest of the Greek army entered and destroyed the city, slaughtering most of the inhabitants.

The story seemed eerily similar to the current situation. It is difficult to read *The Iliad* without thinking how could the Trojans have been so dumb to not check out the horse?! Right? Well, what about us? You'd think we would be a little cautious. BUT NO! We were so happy we had won that no one even questioned whether the Russian's giving up the fight was real. Our defenses were mothballed. Were we making the same mistake?

During the Cold War, the Russians sent "sleepers" into the United States—spies whose mission it was to assimilate themselves into American society before activating and doing damage to the country from within. With the alleged end to the Cold War we forgot about them. What if these sleepers had insinuated themselves so successfully into our society that the Russians called off the frontal assault and pretended to go democratic so that these moles could perform their assignments while we assumed all was well?

I started looking for evidence of assaults on our way of life from within. It's not always easy to distinguish between the actions of foreign spies on the one hand and home grown miscreants on the other. For a long while I was convinced that George W. was a sleeper because it seemed impossible that a real Republican president would devastate the economy by engaging in such massive deficit spending.

However, after painstaking research, I am convinced that the president is not a Russian spy. He's a true, red-blooded American patriot. He just doesn't do very well around numbers. Or words. Or complex problems that require him to think. But hell, he's one of us, and most of us wouldn't do any better.

A lot of people make fun of George W.'s intellect. He may not be a genius, but you can't be dumb and get yourself elected president, even if your brother is governor of the state of Florida and willing to do what is necessary to throw you the state. Heck, it's just one state. No, getting elected if you're a real idiot just doesn't happen. George W. is probably better suited to analyzing facts and making decisions than 99 percent of all Americans. That ain't bad. Of course, if you do the math, that leaves about two to three million Americans who would probably do his job better. Maybe next time we can try one of them.

I gave up looking for spies in politics. Quite frankly, almost all politicians seemed to do things that didn't make sense and that hurt the country. I began looking at everyday life, searching for activity that made no sense and was harmful to our way of life. I had a number of false starts. I was convinced that title insurance companies fit the profile, but it turned out that they were what they seemed on the surface: largely useless companies that charged a lot for doing very little.

Finally, by accident, I hit upon something so arcane that I would not have thought of it in a million years. The criteria fit exactly: it was reducing the quality of life for most Americans and getting worse by the day without reason. I'm talking about product packaging.

I thought of this while trying to take some pills given to me by my doctor. The pills were encased in a package comprised of cardboard with little pockets of plastic attached to the cardboard, in which the pills were contained. You could see the pills; you just couldn't get them out. One was supposed to push the dome until the pills exited through the back of the cardboard, which had been scored to ease the process. Uh huh. There was no way anyone was going to get the pills out that way. I pushed as hard as I could, hurting my fingers and mangling the cardboard. The half domes retained their integrity and kept the pills entrapped. I finally used a knife to extract the pills. Even this wasn't easy.

At first, I was just angry. But then I grew suspicious. Why would anyone package pills that way? It made no sense. Unless…

I investigated the company and learned that they had used a consultant in designing their packaging. The consultant's company had a nondescript name, but when I finally found the individual who had worked on the project, I knew I had struck gold. His first name was Ivan. His second name was an unpronounceable jumble of letters that had no business all being part of a single name. A Ruskie! I got his resumé by pretending to be interested in hiring him. Bingo! He had worked with a veritable Who's Who of American manufacturers, and always on packaging. I reviewed his work and it had a common attribute: all the packaging he designed was absurdly difficult to open.

I began an informal surveillance, and was two weeks into it when something happened. Ivan did what was for him the highly unusual act of going to a bar in the early afternoon. I entered as well, took a seat at the bar, and struck up a conversation. He was extraordinarily dejected, and for the price of buying him more beers than I thought any one man could drink, I was able to get him to tell me the whole story, not only about his mission, but about his childhood, his love life, the unfair way he was being treated by his boss, the different grades of vodka, and so many other things I lost count. I will only summarize the parts about his mission here.

He told me with pride that he had indeed been a Russian spy, a sleeper, but that his mission was over. He had been sent here at the height of the Cold War with directions to work his way into a position where he could help cripple the American economy from within. This is not to say the he needed to do this all by himself; there were others on this assignment as well. It hadn't worked the way he had hoped, and he was being called home by a government that was now concerned that his work would be discovered and cause embarrassment.

Ivan's profession was industrial design; his specialty was packaging— the design and construction of the materials that contained the products we buy. His assignment: make the packaging as difficult as possible to open so that no matter how good the products were, Americans would buy less of them and the American economy would slow down. I was impressed with the diabolical originality of the plot.

Ivan recounted his accomplishments. Most readers are familiar with and regularly curse his work. Have you ever bought a compact disk, or CD, and wondered why it is so hard to open? Thank Ivan. He had found a source of tape that was difficult to see and remove, and worked it into a design that has stood the test of time. The problem, from his point of view, however, was that although people cursed and fumed, they kept buying more and more CDs.

He immediately tackled a variety of other products at the center of the economy. Barbie Dolls and other toys would be broken down into their smallest parts, with each piece then tied securely with metal ties to pieces of cardboard. The ties would then be covered with that invisible and very sticky tape so that you had two challenges rather than one. Again, his hopes were dashed. Although the time to remove a Barbie Doll from its package "improved" from a little under a minute to more than a half an hour, sales were unaffected. Nothing seemed to deter the American consumer from consuming!

He was in the midst of introducing his last and best idea when his recall came. Products would be encased in molded plastic which allowed them to be clearly seen but not touched. At his request, plastic manufacturers introduced new plastics which were incredibly strong and difficult to cut. As an added feature, when one did succeed in cutting it open, the resulting edges would be razor sharp.

I asked him why manufacturers chose these designs rather than ones easier to open. He stared at me for a moment before leaning over and asking me rhetorically in little more than a whisper, "Did you think that I was the only one my country sent over here?" When I realized what he meant and he saw my eyes widen, he continued. "Good lord you people are naïve. I wasn't even the only one working on packaging. We had one fellow who worked with pharmaceuticals. I really admired his plastic bubble attached to thick paper to house pills. I myself have seen desperate people collapse after struggling unsuccessfully to push the pills through the paper. It's great work. I wish it were mine." I told him I was familiar with that one, and agreed that it was a nice piece of work.

I asked him about Styrofoam peanuts. "Yet another team. They were the long range guys. Do you know the half life of that stuff? You will never get rid of it." He sighed. "It's true; the other teams really did much better than I did."

I tried to make him feel better by recounting how many times he had made me miserable. Surely he couldn't be blamed because we Americans bought the products anyway.

"No, my friend," he began, "I have utterly failed. My mission was to deter sales. You Americans are willing to suffer just about anything in order to buy what you want. Who knew there were such people?" With that he gestured to the bartender for another beer. The bartender handed it to him and twisted off the cap in one smooth move. Ivan gave a wry laugh. "You see," he mumbled. "When you really want to, you can make things easy to open. Thank God for that." The beer seemed to lighten his mood. He began singing sad Cossack songs, swaying back and forth with his eyes closed. I decided it was a good time to leave.

Author's Note: At this point, I must do something out of the ordinary and interrupt my own story to confess that it is the work of imagination. While my experiences growing up during the Cold War are all accurately recounted, there is no Russian conspiracy of which I'm aware that has made any efforts to make products more difficult to open. Ivan is an invented personality. I regret having to cut the story short, but we live in a fast moving world where those having the authority to launch air strikes and start wars sometimes act very quickly on allegations without fully checking them out. I didn't want to be responsible for something awful happening before I had a chance to explain that this was satire. Recall the bombers, Mr. President.

But this confession leaves the mystery without an answer: if not some malevolent plot, why do manufacturers seem to favor more and more bizarre packaging? What do they hope to accomplish by making their products so difficult to open?

There is one alternative explanation. It goes by a number of different names in the corporate world—performance gap, lack of customer focus, or stupidity to name a few. The idea is that sometimes people just take their eye off the ball and do a lousy job. It's possible. Based on my experience in the corporate world, it's probable. If that is what is going on, the publicity caused by shining a spotlight on it will have product managers scrambling out of their chairs, calling their subordinates, and telling them they want a full report of their packaging practices and how they were developed by the morning, just in case some executive sees this and wants to know. One thing will lead to another, and companies where it was simply lack of management attention will change their practices and improve their packaging.

If, however, the glare of publicity and management review does not cause a change in practice, then we're back at evil intent. Perhaps I have uncovered something sinister. If I have, we will need to all pitch in and show those Commies that it will never work. How? By shopping like you've never shopped before, buying especially those products whose packaging makes it impossible for you to open them. At my signal!

PART III:

MY BELIEFS

The greatest gift given me by my parents was to allow me to think for myself. Most children are never given the opportunity, but are instead expected to adopt the ideas of their parents. The children's religious instruction is begun before the children are able to grasp that Santa Claus is just a nice story. How can anyone be asked to decide their religious views—which can profoundly affect the rest of their life—at a point when they still believe that the good things in their life are brought by a jolly fat man who (1) lives with elves where it is impossibly cold, (2) visits every home on the planet in a single night to bring the gifts wanted by each child living there, (3) enters each house through the chimney and during the course of a single night consumes several billion cookies and glasses of milk, and (4) is transported from place to place by an old sled pulled by a bunch of reindeer? Granted, the Santa legend is tame compared to some religious beliefs that children are taught to accept as gospel. But the fact that believing in Santa results in a wealth of toys made by elves in China (to whom somebody in the Santa organization obviously outsourced production) is enough of a "believe-stupid-stuff-and get-great-rewards" lesson that no idea proposed by their parents is likely to be challenged.

Imagine instead that a child is told by his parents that he must figure these things out for himself when he is old enough, looking at the world around him to see what makes sense. This is how I was treated, and I believe it gave me an edge over others who looked at the same things I looked at but were able to see only what they had been told they should.

At the very least, I would think that those parents who care whether their children will grow up with the ability to think critically should adopt what I call the "Santa Plus One" rule—that is, don't even begin giving religious, political or other instruction about the beliefs that will carry the child through life until a year after he or she figures out that Santa is just a nice story. The really important things, like treating others with respect and love, the child will absorb anyway, not by reading those words in a book, but hopefully by watching his or her parents live them. If they do not, the words will not help.

I grew up thinking that it was inevitable that I become a lawyer because I argued about everything. I probably took years off my mother's life, and was routinely told by classmates who ran out of other things to say that I was going to go to Hell. As often as not, these predictions were offered during our discussions about evolution, the battle line then and now between scientific thought and religious belief.

There were no laws mandating the teaching of creationism when I was attending Florida public schools. Creationism was taught because the majority of the school board was religious and did not really buy into that nonsense about mankind being descended from monkeys.

The idea that God created man about five thousand years ago was equally silly to me. I had always assumed that when I left Orlando, and lived among less religious people, I would no longer have to defend science against those who believed in the infallibility of ancient texts written by people who sacrificed goats to their God.

I was wrong of course. No less a scientist than George W. Bush has called for renewed debate about evolution in our schools. Creationism, now dressed up as "intelligent design," is making a comeback. There are still hurdles to overcome, such as fossils, carbon dating and other relics of the past, all of which seem to suggest a history a few billion years longer than the biblical accounts permit. No one said this was going to be easy.

There is a museum being built in northern Kentucky that deals with the thorny issue of compressing our planetary history into the biblical timeframes. The common belief of those who take abstractions like carbon dating seriously is that dinosaurs lived millions of years and, fortunately for us, predated man, who came much later. The museum curator does a fabulous job of making the whole thing look more biblically correct by putting a saddle on the dinosaur in the exhibit. Hi-yo triceratops!

Mr. President, I don't want to stifle your nascent interest in education. I also know you owe it to the extremists in your own party to appear as silly as possible when it comes to matters of science. Can we agree that your position on evolution satisfies that obligation fully, and that you will not call for similar debates on whether the Easter bunny exists, or the moon is made of green cheese?

I wish I could be more respectful of our president, but I can't. If he were only silly, that would be okay. But he matches his Winnie-the-Bush status (a president of little brain) with an arrogant assuredness that he is right, a deadly combination for many others. Having Parkinson's disease, and suffering directly from his decision to block promising medical research on religious grounds, it is difficult not to see red when I think of him.

Ironically, the fact that he *is* Winnie the Bush is the best evidence supporting the notion that Darwin may have been wrong or at least too simplistic. If the president is no brighter than I and other "liberals" think, how is it that he exists this many millions of years into the evolutionary game of Survivor? God may choose to create dummies for his own reasons; evolution is not supposed to.

Fifth Interlude:

The Origins of Idiots

It's a little late in the day to revisit the debate over evolution. Darwin's theory, summarized bloodily and briefly as the "survival of the fittest," is now accepted by most rational people as fact. Fossils are sold at natural history museums. People even have warmed to the notion that we share common ancestry with primordial slime. It helps explain some of their relatives. Evolution has become comfortable because it proves what we want to believe—that we are the best, that after hundreds of millions of years of creatures and entire species losing out in the battle to survive, it is we who are kings and queens of the mountain!

Yet something is wrong. I finally was able to identify what was troubling me after spending the day with representatives of a large insurance company, trying to secure their necessary pre-approval to obtain medical treatment for my wife. These were not the truly smart but evil types who squashed the hopes of the few insured who broke through the early skirmish lines. These were the early greeters, whose job it was to be very pleasant but use their innate lack of intelligence to thin the claimant ranks by answering each question incorrectly and sending claimants the wrong forms. With evolution culling the imperfect from the herd, where did the insurance companies find such people? Or to put the question generically:

If humans endured millions of years of evolutionary struggle from which only the fittest could emerge, why are we surrounded by morons?

It's not an easy question. Evolution has been going on for a very long time, with the unfit being eaten or otherwise rendered non-procreative. The ancestors of the current batch of idiots couldn't have been too sharp either, so why did they live to sire progeny rather than ending up in the belly of a large prehistoric crocodile? Something was not quite right with Darwin's thinking.

I heard in the background an account of a baseball game. The Yankees, with the best line-up that money could buy, were losing to a lesser team. It took me a minute to realize the significance of this to evolutionary theory. Sometimes the best team didn't win! The fittest should, but did not always, win out! Darwin had overlooked probability theory.

The most enjoyable illustration of probability theory is the truism that if there are enough monkeys sitting at enough typewriters, it is probable that one monkey will type, if only by happy accident, a Shakespearean sonnet. Don't try this at home. It requires a very large number of monkeys. Even if you did round up enough, think of the feeding, the other bodily functions, the public health clearances and so on. What a mess. This helps explain why Shakespeare remains so famous despite his sometimes awkward phrasing—he could write those same sonnets without the monkeys, allowing him to produce great art at low cost and without a lot of fuss.

It's only fitting to apply this monkey story to evolution. Darwin assumed that the fittest would survive and prosper. They should, but occasionally the fittest just have a bad day. Now think of probability theory playing out through the expanse of the universe on the untold number of planets where fit and unfit do battle. If, as appears likely, we are dealing with as many planets as Shakespeare-wannabee monkeys, then the same improbable results would probably occur on some of those planets. Just as most monkeys would type gibberish, some would type a few insipid words, and every once in a long while one would type a Shakespearean sonnet, so on most planets the fittest would survive, on a few it would be a mixed bag, and on some planet somewhere the least fit would consistently survive and reproduce.

Think of an African plain where a hungry lion is stalking a herd of gazelles. Picture two gazelles. The first is a bucktoothed misfit with one foot shorter than the rest, resulting in a limp and a lack of speed out of the blocks. The other gazelle is buff and knows it, with bulging leg muscles toned by constant sprints, capable of blinding speed, and possessing a scent that drives female gazelles wild. On virtually every one of the millions and millions of planets, the name and picture of the second gazelle will appear in the family tree.

On that planet of the long odds where sonnets are written, the buff gazelle steps in a gopher hole and traps his foot. His last coherent thought as the lion's bite forces him to lose consciousness is disbelief that bucktooth is trotting away into the area of bush popular for gazelle procreation with a nubile female. Repeat the improbable enough times, generation after generation, and you will have a planet on which only the least fit survive. Mr. Darwin studied animals, not the stars, and he likely had no thoughts about other planets where lions may chase gazelles. Darwinism needs to be refined to acknowledge that on most planets the most fit will survive, while at the extreme end of improbability there will be a planet on which only the least fit survive, and stretched out in between will be an array of planets where, to varying degrees, the most fit should but occasionally don't survive.

What kind of planet are we on? Misfits seem to be thriving, and the fit seem in increasing peril. The thought depressed me. I closed my papers and started to stand up, having no more energy to fight the forces of evil that day. As I did so, I felt a gentle tug at my sleeve by someone trying to rouse my attention. It was one of the insurance greeters with my insurance coverage forms in his hands. He looked puzzled. "They've been approved," he said. "You, know," he added, "I can't remember that ever happening before. Oh you hear stories, but to actually see coverage approved. Wow!" Thoughts of going home empty handed vanished. I had my insurance!

The greeter went over to some of his friends to tell of his participation in this rare event. They soon went off to tell others, and I was left unsupervised. I looked at the door from which the greeter had emerged with news of my coverage. The impulse was irresistible. I opened the door wanting to see and perhaps even thank him or her. I was shocked to see row after row of monkeys sitting before typewriters, denying insurance applications.

As I stared with my mouth hanging open, I noticed one monkey, wearing what looked to be an old Jerry Garcia tie, smiling at me. I'll be damned if he didn't wink. I don't know if he'll ever type a sonnet, but he did enough that day to earn a place on the mountain. I winked back, and left to share the unexpectedly good news with my wife.

Evolution remains one of the most fascinating ideas to explore. Why not? It is the byproduct of mating selection (sexual attraction) and survival (violence), the two themes on which most modern culture is based. Liberals tend to focus on the first input (sexual attraction) while criticizing those who focus on the second. Conservatives, of course, are more comfortable talking about killing than about sex. As an open-minded writer, I have explored both in the next two Interludes. The first deals with the male fascination with the female breast; the second, with the consequences of modern man's escape from the Darwinian cycle of violence.

Exploring such topics, particularly when it touches such sensitive topics as why our bodies are the way they are, may offend some. I count women with large breasts among my friends. I know how tiresome it is for them to be stared at for this reason and how large breasts may affect comfort and health. I confess an almost adolescent fascination with this part of their anatomy, and must acknowledge that I am more attracted to their breasts than their elbows. I wrote this not to make them feel uncomfortable, but to search for an explanation of why that is.

Sixth Interlude:

The Origins of Women with Large Breasts

I was dining in the Ryland Inn, an expensive New Jersey restaurant, when I was struck by one of those mathematical relationships that remind one of the underlying majesty of nature. Though observable and observed by all, but especially by men, what I am about to describe is not yet the subject of scholarly dissertation. I startled my two male companions who had been struggling to eat their oysters with their jaws hanging open, by stating the issue before us as follows:

"There is a statistically significant relationship between the price of the entrees on a restaurant menu and the breast size of the women dining there."

Having tumbled to this through the observation of a particularly compelling example, I would have been content to relax, drink wine, and spend the evening refining my observations. My friends, however, knew of my passion for Darwinian analytics and asked me to either explain myself or to stop trying to confuse science and beauty. In other words, could I just shut up and enjoy the view? I thought for a moment only, and told them this was too important to ignore. One of them ordered another bottle of wine, which I thought was a tremendous gesture, so I began.

The fact that rich men, that is, men who could have everything, liked women with large breasts concealed a rich web of underlying evolutionary riddles. Women with large breasts have evolved and have thrived. Why? Men are attracted to women with large breasts. Why again? Finally, why were these large-breasted women attracted to men with money, or at least willing to dine with them?

I know at this point a few readers will think this is less scientific than they had expected, and other readers will be mortified by my assumption that the men in attendance had the money and the women in attendance were the objects of pursuit. I mean no offense to either group, and certainly do not intend any unseemly titillation. This is science. I will keep the discussion dry and to the point, but I must follow where the evidence leads and cannot avoid the facts simply because they may be socially offensive.

Conan Doyle said that if you eliminate the impossible, what remains, however improbable, will be the truth. Let's start with why big-breasted women have survived. One can eliminate the possibility that babies of big-breasted women survive more frequently and therefore propagate that gene more successfully. Babies need just enough of a grip to get a good feed and that's not much. No evidence exists that they get any boost from breast size beyond that. As a matter of fact, it is likely that some infants may not have survived the consequences of feedings by excessively endowed mothers who dozed off during the experience. If anything, the nod from the infants' camp would be in favor of small breasts.

Nor does available evidence support that large-breasted women survive and reach reproductive age more successfully than their smaller-breasted peers. Looking back on the millions of years when the game of survivor was going on in earnest, women with large breasts would have been a step slower then those with more streamlined torsos. I'm not saying women with large breasts can't run. They can and they should. Larger breasts are a hindrance to evasive maneuvers, however, and women with larger breasts likely would have been caught more frequently by predators.

If larger breasts were not helpful for woman or child, the higher mortality rates of those with this physiology must have been over-compensated by higher rates of reproduction by those who did survive. Why did our prehistoric forefathers go for well-endowed cave women? Definitions of beauty are not carved in stone, yet this male inclination must have a long and ancient history.

Darwin would have had an answer, but given that he was long dead, I proudly provided one that I thought he would have liked. Assuming that at one point in our history men pursued women of all breast sizes indifferently, mutations in man's brain created a craving to impregnate women with nice round breasts more than women with no breasts or breasts that had lost their fight with gravity. Those with this mutation must have produced more offspring than others, resulting in the evolution of men who think of reproducing themselves when they see a woman with a bountiful bosom.

It makes sense. Women who had large and uplifted breasts, at least in our prehistoric history, were more likely to be fertile than those with either very small breasts (who might have been too young) or with less uplifted breasts (who might have been too old) to reproduce. Those males who were genetically engineered to pursue the shapely breasted females were thus more likely to reproduce and perpetuate this genetic trait in their male descendants. This realization holds the promise for better understanding between the sexes. Men who stare at women's breasts are not boors. They are merely acting out their genetic programming to preserve the species by looking for the sort of curve that nature has made men, unconsciously, recognize as a sign to disrobe and fight for human survival.

That explains the male behavior. I was about to tackle the mystery of female attraction to men with money when I was brought to an abrupt halt by my colleagues who had grown weary of science. My friend to my right took a deep drink of his wine, looked at the original subject of my curiosity, and with one comment evidenced his lack of interest in further explanation: "Ah," he said, "they're probably not real anyway."

I was stunned into silence. I tried to remember my wife's advice as to how to tell real from unreal when he continued. "You know," he said with a wry smile, "this simply proves that the jury is still out as to whether Darwin's violent theories are really more accurate than the gentle science of Lamarck." The name was disturbingly familiar, and I struggled to remember something, anything. I needn't have.

"Jean Baptiste Lamarck," he continued, "based his evolutionary theory on two laws: first, that frequent and sustained use of any organ 'strengthens that organ, develops and enlarges it,' and second, that such traits, once acquired are passed down to subsequent generations. Now, while the examples he used were things like a blacksmith's arm, take a look again at the lovely lady. Can you imagine her breasts getting any less use than a blacksmith's arm? Not likely. Even if they're not real, the motivation to have them enlarged—to cause greater use—seems decidedly more Lamarckian than Darwinian."

After some moments spent looking like a guppy that had accidentally leapt from its bowl, I was about to assert that Lamarck was an idiot and that use of one's breasts did not increase their size. Even that pathetic response was muted by the sudden appearance at our table of the beauty who had started it all. Glowering at me, she said in a tone normally used with unruly school children, "Do you have nothing better to do than stare at a woman's breasts and talk nonsense? If your friend didn't have such a nice smile, I would have asked that you be told to leave."

She shifted her eyes to my friend, her glance changing from withering to warming as she swiveled to look at him. With a smile, she finished, "As for you, I would love to meet you and see whether there is anything to Lamarck's theories." With that they began some sort of information exchange accompanied by winks, nods, and an occasional scornful look in my direction.

Holding to Darwin as a life raft, I struggled home and crawled into bed, waiting for the mercy of sleep. I closed my eyes, and hoped that the new day would prove that this had all been a bad dream.

☆ ☆ ☆

Those who abhor violence have missed a vital fact about humanity. It is why we are here. If we were not the best killers on the planet, some other species would be harvesting *us*. We have so curtailed the presence of violence in our lives that the *Pax Homo Sapiens* may in fact jeopardize our future existence. I'm not condoning wars or terrorism; those forms of violence do nothing to further the species' interests because those engaging in such activity normally use non-evolutionary criteria to target their victims.

Without predators picking off the less fit, we have created an enviable position where all members of the species can experience the joys of parenthood. That's wonderful. The question that becomes worrisome is whether that is stable. Other species are continuing to evolve, and it is likely unless something changes that we will lose our dominant position sometime in the future.

I have a deep-rooted fear of insects, especially roaches. I see in their vast numbers and their ability to lose huge portions of their population to pesticides only to have the survivors replenish their ranks with equal numbers of resistant super-bugs, the seeds of future peril for humanity. True, they have not yet become aggressive in most cases, and we derive great comfort from that. What will happen when they do?

SEVENTH INTERLUDE:
THE FUTURE OF THE SPECIES

We and every other species compete with each other for galactic domination. Thus far we're doing very well. We are the unquestioned masters of all we see, and we demonstrate our preeminence in the accepted ways of victors—by using the skins of the vanquished to make gloves and shoes, by turning others into soap, and by eliminating some species altogether if they happen to get too familiar.

Being so far ahead of the next closest contender masks a fundamental weakness. We are no longer evolving, while those species with which we compete are. We have created a protective cocoon around ourselves so that all humans can survive and reproduce, whether or not they would under the harsher rule of Mother Nature. We do not really compete for survival with other species. Where we have contests with other species, the contest is rigged to make certain that the human combatant emerges the winner.

In our games of survival with animals, for example, humans get high powered rifles and camouflage, and the animals get, well, nothing. Intra-species competitions are generally designed to be non-fatal as well. Outside of Latin America, for instance, losers of athletic contests are rarely executed. Even where human competitions are designed to be fatal, the selection process for elimination is indiscriminate rather than selective. Wars don't target weaker members of the herd; they kill at random, seemingly often taking the best among us, leaving us individually poorer and collectively stagnant.

Not so with our competition. Other species continue to get slaughtered by the tens of thousands or by the millions at the hands of traditional predators and by man, the evolutionary accelerator. The carnage makes those species better and better. While our lead over our competition is substantial, our stagnation and their continued improvement will result in competing species overtaking us and achieving domination. That is a frightening thought. Will that species harvest humans for something found desirable to that species? Suppose they decided one small but critical piece of our bodies is fashionable to wear or is an aphrodisiac? Could any species be so heartless?

Allow me to present a relatively benign example of what could easily be our future.

Many of you are familiar with what we see as "the deer problem." In New Jersey and many other areas of the Northeast, an overabundance of these sweet-faced animals in human population areas has led to widespread carnage on the roads. Deer are constantly stumbling into the paths of cars. Is it my imagination, or are the survivors getting smarter?

If not today then soon, their behavior will cease being explained by "deer in the headlights" stupidity, and instead morph into calculated efforts to drive humans from their habitat. Although there are no known link-ages between the groups, the deer tactics are not unlike many other terrorist groups launching suicide attacks on those they oppose. How long will it take evolution to produce uber-deer who have the abilities to transform this disorganized mayhem into an organized jihad? How will we cope with malevolent deer leaders bent on a deer homeland once they discover plastic explosives?

In the deepest part of the forest, the uber-deer whine about the lack of intelligent troops while using stories about pretty does slaughtered by hunters to generate hundreds and thousands of deer volunteers ready to strap on explosives and die for a deer homeland! What else have these villainous animals been up to? Is Jimmy Hoffa really buried under Giant Stadium as has been popularly rumored, or is he being held by deer terrorists in a POW camp somewhere beyond the edges of civilization?

Without admitting that we would ever negotiate with terrorists, one can imagine that we might need to cede land to buy peace. If we could limit the losses, say, to eastern New Jersey, that might be tolerable, but we might be forced to give up something of real value. If the uber-deer are smart, as they would need to be, can we really have any comfort that they would settle for the Interstate 95 corridor?

I am not trying to be melodramatic. If I really wanted to frighten you, I would not have talked about deer. Think about cockroaches and the risks of a human-insect conflict with humans unimproved and the insects a few billion generations into the future. Those sneaky bastards would start the conflict despite early attempts to accommodate them. Florida would be lost for sure, and the humans who survived would end up in slave camps making cardboard.

What is the solution? I think moving backwards to re-join the Darwinian process would be politically unpalatable. We graduated from that unpleasant phase of evolution and would not want to return. Would the public support preventing those of our young who were slow at school, awkward at sports and so forth from reproducing themselves? Any politician who even raised the idea would face certain political ruin.

We need a new evolutionary vehicle that allows humanity to continue to improve despite our graduation from Darwinism. We must move from Darwin's Law of Natural Selection to what I refer to as the Law of Improved Selection.

I was doing other important research at a bar in St. Thomas called Duffy's Love Shack when the solution struck me. The female attendees who appeared interested in reproductive activities were pursuing males whose main claim to fame appeared to be really neat tattoos and the occasional ability to express words of two syllables. "Natural Selection" was not going to produce an improved next generation this way.

I became troubled solely because of the implications this had on the future of mankind. Humanity's evolutionary progress depends almost entirely on the mating selections made by the female. We males think that our job is to try to impregnate everything that moves, or looks like it may move in the foreseeable future. I am not defending our behavior, I am merely describing it and offering an opinion that to pin hopes on males declining to mate with any willing female is like going to the racetrack and betting the future of humanity on a blind horse with a broken leg.

Unfortunately, the females of our species have been little more selective than the males. Because so much depends on their using judgment at a moment when they're not thinking too clearly, the following guidelines, which they could study in advance, should help improve their choice of male breeding partners:

1. Discard partners who use in the first sentence they utter "hey babe," "hey baby" or any other witticism that suggests an inability to think above the waist.

2. One tattoo could have been a mistake; two or more indicate knowing disfigurement. Discard immediately. (Note: This, like the other rules, is only intended to apply to males. We recognize that there are very attractive women who sport classy tattoos. We do not mean to be critical of such things; indeed we mean no criticism of anything done by very attractive women. You can play the accordion to your heart's

content, have tattooed butterflies on your butts, and have silly laughs. I don't want to be unfairly judgmental.)

3. Body piercing doesn't get the benefit of the one free strike rule; if a man does this, he's out.

4. Do they like accordion? Out. Wayne Newton? Out. Mahler? Out. If they don't love Mozart, Chopin, Beethoven, the Beatles and the Rolling Stones, they are out as well.

5. If they think wrestling is a sport, or majored in political science, it's best to decline their genetic contributions. Our model predicts steady improvement of our position vis a vis other species if those with these attributes do not contribute to the gene pool.

6. Short men are out. We don't need more humans with Napoleon complexes.

7. Men who sound like a hyena when they laugh are gone.

8. Men who bray like a donkey during intimacy are also out, but since this discovery may be made too late to help in individual cases, it is incumbent on females to add this to the list of male traits during intimacy they already share with other females.

9. Men who talk about God and the divine mission they have been asked to perform are out, but can be re-qualified if it turns out they have one.

10. Finally, men who have not bought a copy of this book will be given one chance to buy it, but are out if they fail to do so. Those who wish to contribute to the gene pool must recognize truth and beauty when placed right in front of their noses.

While not perfect, these criteria certainly seem better than the criteria used by women today. Ladies, may we get started? I remind you the alternatives are not pretty.

PART IV:

Coming of Age

Beatrice Lefer, my mother, was an intelligent and beautiful woman who did not pursue education beyond high school because her family was poor. Her father, never a business success, died while she was young, and it was necessary for her to begin working so that her younger brother could get an education. That's the way it was.

She died in November 2004. She shaped my life and the lives of my brother and sister so completely that it is sometimes difficult to accept that she is really gone. In some ways she is still here. I have a picture of her that I hung near the dining table in our home. When my father was staying with me he used to look at that picture every time I offered dessert. Nine times out of ten, he would then say no, telling me "she wouldn't have liked it if I did."

They were married forty-nine and a half years and would have made fifty and beyond but for her death. They were an old fashioned couple in many ways. My father took responsibility for making a living, and my mother stayed home and raised the children. Although the woman's movement raised questions about the fairness of this arrangement, it like everything else is what you make of it. Beatrice turned her life, and ours, into a rich treasure-trove of experiences so that I think it was my father, though uncommonly successful in his career, who was short-changed.

That is not to say our upbringing was without its problems. My mother was over-protective and stubborn as a mule. I was stubborn as two mules. It made for some interesting clashes. I remember the aftershocks of one of our arguments, though I have no recollection what it was we had argued about. During the course of the exchange I said something that she felt crossed the line. I would not apologize because I was convinced, as always, that I was right. She imposed what was for her a severe punishment: I would watch no television until I apologized.

I was banned from television for over a year, but still would not apologize. It was she who finally withdrew the banishment, allowing me to watch some show with the rest of the family while saying words that turned out to be prophetic, "I just hope you marry someone who can put up with you!" I'm not proud of this outcome, and I wish I had apologized. I offer this story to explain why I am the way I am, not to brag about it.

Besides, while I have been unsuccessful at marriage, my daughter's dog loves me.

Eighth Interlude:
About My Mother

I grew up in an extremely tight knit family, and my family helped shape much of my personality. My way of looking at things logically was a result of my father teaching me math and chess. My creative side resulted from trying to survive my mother's conversion to health foods.

Eating healthy foods is good but boring. Coping with someone who has embraced health foods as a way of life is another matter. For a child who dreamt of ice cream, Hershey bars and candied popcorn, it was a struggle for the things that made life itself worthwhile. I fought to avoid having what I ate control what I did. I remember the request to spend the night at a friend's house:

Q: "Can I go spend the night at Billy's? His mother said it was okay." Billy was really cool and this visit would immediately raise my stature at school.

A: "No, you know that you can't. They don't eat healthy and I'm not going to have you eat junk."

Q: "Well then, can he come over here? His mom said that would be okay too." I had done my homework. This time I thought I had her in a corner.

A: "No. Billy wouldn't enjoy what we eat, and besides, if he came over here, they would expect you to go over there, and I don't want you to do that because you would eat junk."

Game, set and match.

I should confess one inaccuracy in the reference to her as "my mother." More accurately, she was "our mom." I have an older brother and sister. Yet, while our experiences were similar, mine hit at a younger age. When wonderful chocolate was banished from our house and replaced with that most insidious, foul-tasting imposter, carob, my brother and sister were older and had enjoyed chocolate birthday cakes for most of their formative years. Not I.

I was eleven years old and becoming more anxious about social acceptance, when my mother surprised me at my birthday party by bringing out a carob birthday cake. She of course promised that it would be "just as good" as the chocolate ones she had made previously. One taste was enough to convince me that I was going to gag and die. Even if I didn't, my friends would all be convinced that I had known about this and led them into a trap where they would gag and die.

How could a woman who was so warm and loving be transformed into Attila the Hun when it came to food? You think I exaggerate? Let's start with breakfast. One cannot mention the word in my family without two feared words coming to mind—egg drink. That was the concoction made daily by my mother for which we could have had her hauled away for abuse. It was made with a raw egg base, into which would be poured all sorts of healthy powders —dolomite, carob, calcium, or frankly anything that had received a favorable write-up in *Prevention* magazine. This was then mixed together in a blender with water, or milk if the latter was starting to go bad. It produced a brown-looking drink, with a brackish head of foam. It chilled the soul to look at it, and scarred the soul to drink it.

My mother always was looking to improve it. In fact, our liberation from egg drinks came the day she decided to add the egg shells along with the eggs, in order to increase the calcium content. Why not? It would all go through the blender. The usual decibel level at the breakfast table went off the charts, and my mother finally agreed to taste her own drink to see what all the fuss was about. She immediately pronounced it undrinkable and asked in complete and maddening sincerity why we had never said something about it.

The idea of a breakfast drink itself wasn't bad. We had to have something to wash down the vitamins we consumed. We had over a hundred a day. My personal record was swallowing seventeen at one time, but my sister topped me, emptying a Dixie cup nearly full of pills into her mouth, which she downed with an orange juice chaser.

I should mention before we move to lunch that this all happened in the 1960s, before health foods had really hit the big time. My mother was a pioneer and was probably one of the first to read Rachel Carson's great book *Silent Spring* about the overuse of chemicals. She approached diet with a religious fervor, and she didn't give a hoot what others might think.

Which brings us to lunch. That was the worst meal of the day because, as a teenager, I did care what others thought of me. How lucky the kids were who were allowed to purchase their lunches at school and blend in with everyone else! It was a little awkward to bring a lunch, but you could get away with it if it was cool stuff, wrapped in some simple aluminum foil or something. You were lost at sea, though, if you showed up as I did with a large brown bag packed with one freakish looking thing after another.

Bread should be flexible. Most is. Well, my mom made her own dark brown bread, sometimes with virtually no flour, and it did not bend. If you got it the first day or two after it was made, it crumbled into a million little pieces when you bit it. It was like a building collapsing. The sandwich infrastructure would crumble into your hands, followed by the one to two pounds of meat or other ingredients that had temporarily been placed in between the slices.

After the second day, I would remember wistfully when mere teeth could put a dent in the bread. It would become so hard that you could only hope to take a bite by putting your full weight and strength into the effort. Generally this didn't work. When it did, the breakthrough would be so violent that the sandwich contents would end up exploding into the air. This was just the sort of display a teenage boy did not want to make of himself during the part of the day when others were acting cool and pursuing their hormonal instincts free of such embarrassment.

Dinner was special. It was a time when the family assembled together almost without fail. My father would come home for family dinner, even though he would have to work after we went to bed. We were expected not to be off with friends. Our dinners frequently were blessed with wonderful food as well. My mother was a great cook when she allowed herself to be, and she cooked meats and made salads with such skill that it would make your mouth water. But there were also those dark days of chicken liver and broccoli. No waste was tolerated, so we sat at the table until done. In rare cases, when I was still at the table well after bedtime, my mother would feel sorry for me and permit me to go to bed, provided I promised to finish what was left for breakfast. It sounds worse than it was; given that the alternative to eating your leftover dinner was an egg drink, this wasn't all bad.

I wasn't brave enough to enjoy being different. Teenagers like to fit in, not explain why they seem weird. I had no choice. My diet forced me to use humor and creativity to try to come up with reasons why I wasn't as strange as I seemed on the surface. It didn't matter that I didn't succeed. It was the practice that taught me to think fast, think differently, and to use humor as a defense. I am not suggesting that you do this to your own kids, but it's something to think about.

Food was merely a vehicle used by my mother to keep us glued tightly together. While I resented its use as a wall to keep others out, I now recognize the magic of using something, anything, to keep tight bonds within. In addition to strange food, my mother dished out love and interest in us in portions so large that they would fit comfortably into a Dickens novel. There was a total commitment to our well-being that seemed so natural, but was in fact exceptional. Even now, I am not surprised when my mother, who suffers more than I from the ravages of age and health, looks at me with loving eyes and tells me she would give anything if she could have my Parkinson's disease afflict her rather than me.

I sometimes sit beside her when I visit and make her laugh and smile. I can get away with a lot now, because her body has betrayed her, despite all that health food, and she cannot smack me. Despite her health problems and her oft-expressed desire to not continue living in her present condition, she refuses to eat anything but health foods. She is willing to travel thirty minutes to a pizza parlor solely because it uses whole wheat crusts, passing along the way about three or four hundred pizza places that make pizza far better.

When I look back on these experiences with the benefits of age, I realize the importance of her actions had little to do with food. Instead, what I will remember is a love so strong that it caused her to torture us with what she thought was best.

Postscript: This once vital and vibrant woman died November 10, 2004, after a long convalescence following a stroke. I have a marvelous mental image of her in Heaven, sitting and watching her children and grandchildren playing on Earth below. She is wearing her favorite forty-year-old bathrobe, covering a shirt I wore to summer camp as a teenager. She has a candy bar in her hand, and there are more candy wrappers on the floor. She is saying to God between mouthfuls, "Why didn't you let me know that sugar was Your true gift to mankind? Boy, this is good. Gabriel, can you pass that box of M&Ms?"

Don't worry about a thing. Pop will do fine. This week we're showing him pictures of pots and pans and explaining when they were invented and what they're used for. He's shown some interest in the cast iron skillet and said with some basic re-design work, nothing fancy, it could be turned into a very useful tool for housing nuclear devices. As for food, you don't need to worry: each day we visit a different fast food establishment. Burger King is the current front runner because Pop liked their fries better than Wendy's, but this is a crazy world where anything can happen.

Goodbye. I will cherish my memories of you as long as I live.

I have few regrets about my childhood. I will mention only two, neither of which is worth mentioning more than in a fleeting way. The first is that, having had a dog as an adult, I realize how much I missed having one as a child. I didn't have one because I was the youngest, and my sister already had dashed any hopes either my brother or I might have harbored for pets of our own by exhausting our parents' tolerance for pets. She had parakeets. You're probably thinking of one or two birds kept in a cute little parakeet cage. No, I'm talking about more than a dozen of those winged creatures, unrestrained by the bars of any cage. They were birds, for crying out loud, not criminals!

My sister had a big heart. Each time she went to a pet store, she would come home with a new bird or two, rescued because (she claimed) they looked either unhappy or unhealthy in the cages there. Though she had a cage in her room the size of a whale, she felt no less sorry for them if they were locked up there. After wearing my parents down, she finally won the right to allow them to fly about out of the cage so long as they stayed in her room. Every once in a while, when someone would take too long opening or closing her door, one of the parakeets would escape and the chase would be on throughout the house!

Though I did not think it was fair, I really could not blame my mother for limiting my brother and me afterwards to tropical fish. These were frustrating pets. You could not do anything with them, they never smiled or acted as if they wanted to be with you, and they seemed to live only a short time.

That is close to being an accurate description for my relationships with women, my second regret. I was a painfully shy young man made to feel like an outsider because of my religious beliefs, my food habits and my family. I pursued nerdish hobbies such as chess and classical piano, and though I was very aware of girls, I was totally inept and had no idea of how to get close to them. My relationships with females were early Woody Allen—the nerd with glasses who made a total fool of himself in the presence of any woman (or girl) to whom he was attracted. Somewhere along the line Woody Allen's persona changed, and the story focused on him screwing things up and losing a woman that he had.

I emulated his early period—you can't lose what you never had. Frustrated, I lashed out at my nerdness. I retired from competitive chess at the age of sixteen. It took a while, but I finally noticed that there were no females frequenting the tables at the Orlando Chess Club Friday nights. Playing each Friday till midnight sharpened my game, but to what end? So, despite having made a brief pre-retirement appearance in the list of the top twenty-five players in the country under the age of sixteen, and despite what could have been satisfying wins over two master-level opponents in tournament play, I gave it up, bought a pair of bell-bottom pants, and went out on a date.

The sixties might have explained the shape of the pants I wore, though not well. The times merely provided outlets for bad taste; they did not require that you pick the bad over the good that was also available. Nor did they explain my color choice. The closest I can come to describing it is the word "turquoise." I am horrified but am also compelled to add that there were pinstripes involved. I cannot honestly remember what thinking, what perverse self-destructive logic, guided me to buy those pants, and afterwards, to wear them.

My date took one look at me when she opened the front door of her parents' house and announced that she had to be back by 10 pm. We had planned to go to a movie that ended 20 minutes before that, allowing just enough time to drive her home without stops. With my failure decreed up front, the downward spiral of the evening was at least not a surprise.

I began to focus on college as the place where I would fix my lack of social skills and achieve social success. I did not share my criteria for choosing a college with my parents for obvious reasons. My father was puzzled and a bit disappointed when I turned down the opportunity to study physics at his alma mater (Cooper Union) to study philosophy at Boston University. I had wanted to be a lawyer since I was a kid, and I needed to have an undergraduate degree first. Philosophy was as good as physics for that. Besides, when you study philosophy as an undergraduate in Boston, you have time for other things.

NINTH INTERLUDE:

FRIENDS FOR LIFE

Thirty-five years ago, I left home to attend college. I was innocent and under-educated, so I picked a school in Boston, Massachusetts, that seemed capable of curing both conditions. That first year I made little progress on either, and at the time I would have told you that the year was a disappointment.

I now realize I had been judging the year incorrectly. I may not have met the goals I had then, but I began friendships that dwarfed in importance what I thought I wanted. My friendships with three individuals I met that year—John, David and Fred—have been the most enduring friendships of my life. These friendships have grown strong as a result of the experiences we have shared over the last three decades, and I am confident that they will last my lifetime.

The Curious Case of the Bowling Alley Goddess. Then (being 1970) and now, Boston had a large number of unattached females. Many were pretty, some were beautiful, but the Bowling Alley Goddess was the perfect embodiment of sexuality, fantasy and feminine beauty in one unbelievable woman. She had curves where they were supposed to be, sparkling eyes, a captivating smile, and an abundance of those features that make men who love women remember why they do.

You probably think I am exaggerating. If anything, I fail to do her justice. On a scale of one to ten, she was at least a twenty. Here John and I were, stupid little freshmen who had just met and had gone bowling for something to do, and she was in the lane next to us! She was nice as well, and talking to us in a very unaffected and open way.

You've heard of deer-in-the-headlights stupidity. Deer are dim-witted animals that, though fully capable of avoiding most cars, seem sometimes to freeze in the face of danger and get run over. We made them look decisive.

I, of course, had an excuse. Her smile, when she bestowed it on us, had melted the soles of my shoes and I was stuck to the floor. Besides, though I hate to admit it, she was more interested in my friend John. This really wasn't that surprising. Fate had decreed that John would be more handsome in the early years and I in the later. I can't remember when the crossover point is to occur, but it should be soon! This was John's opportunity, and I assign him full responsibility for what happened.

John was able to break from his stupor sufficiently to utter a few words to the Goddess. For a moment she thought she had a live one. As I recall, his opening line was well constructed and avoided biting off more than he could chew. I think it was: "Are you a student here too?" A solid start! Sadly, he had exhausted his stock of courage with this forceful beginning, and he began to stammer and wither before her beautiful eyes. Her face was expressive as well as beautiful, and I was able to watch as it reflected first disappointment, then frustration, and then a desire to escape. I have experienced much sadness in my life, but few things have matched the feeling of utter emptiness as this perfect beauty left the bowling alley a short while later and walked out of our lives.

Shared humiliation is fertile soil for lasting friendship. This was only the first of many humbling experiences. With each experience, the bonds among the four of us grew stronger. Given our sustained poor performance during the entire first year, we built a foundation for friendship strong enough to last our lifetimes. It's odd to think that the social success we wanted more than anything would have diverted us from the task of building that foundation and weakened the bonds of lasting friendship. At the time we would have made the trade in an instant, but now I'm grateful for our ineptitude.

Following the end of freshman year, we went our separate ways. I dropped out of college to travel the world. My parents were not impressed and made it clear that I should behave responsibly (i.e., stay in school) if I wanted continued financial support. Feeling the invulnerability of youth, I had a great year traveling, and finished my undergraduate degree at University of Florida, where the in-state tuition was about what I now pay for cable television service. I earned enough during the summer to pay for tuition and living expenses the following year. College finished, parents placated, I headed back to Boston for law school.

The House on the Hill. Once I knew I was going back to Boston, I got in touch with John and asked if he knew of a place to stay. He lived in a group house in Brookline, which happened to have a vacancy. For just under $60 a month, I had a home.

The house was a blight on an otherwise nice neighborhood. Though modest, the neighborhood was filled with people who had pride in themselves and their homes. All the other houses were well cared for. The yards were attractive and well kept, with colorful gardens. Then there was our house. It was a rental, not cared for at all by the owner and only fitfully maintained by us when we were both sober and bored. That didn't happen very often. In our defense, we *were* college students.

I am certain the neighbors hated us. The paint on our house was peeling, and the few blades of grass in the yard had long ago surrendered to the weeds, which then began creeping towards the unspoiled beauty of the neighbors' lawns. The outside wasn't much, but at least it prevented what was inside from spilling into view. You think you know what a messy house is like? Multiply the worst you've ever seen by two or three. True, there are a lot of talented amateurs out there. We were professionals, and among us, Fred was the best.

Fred Bread and Cottism. Fred was and is one of a kind. He lived in a crook in a hallway where we had been able to squeeze in a collapsible cot at a slant. Fred had an elegant yet simple approach to life that would have been much admired by Thoreau: during the day he put his possessions on the cot; at night when he wanted to use the cot, he put them underneath. I have become convinced over time that this approach towards life offers a chance for happiness greater than most religions.

At the right time, I intend to start a movement called "Cottism," based on Fred's embellishment of Thoreau's original work. I am reluctant to do it now, however, because after years of dedicated bachelorhood, Fred appears to have found his soul mate, Connie. I worry about the impact his deification will have on their relationship. I also want to delay this until I no longer have a Porsche. I think you can reconcile Thoreau with having a Porsche, but why give your critics an easy target?

No mention of Fred would be complete without a reference to what we called "Fred bread." I was surprised at how good it was given the casual approach Fred took in making it. He would walk around the house using a wooden spoon to mix the dough, occasionally putting the bucket he used as a mixing bowl down to pursue some other interest. The bucket may have held the secret to the bread. Fred never cleaned it. He simply scraped out the major pieces of crusted remains from the previous session when he was ready to make another few loaves.

Good bakers use something called "biga" or starter dough to enhance the flavor of the bread. It is dough carefully cared for from an earlier batch. Fred took this well beyond traditional thinking. The resulting bread was delightful—probably among the best breads I've ever had. I realize as I write this that I have not tasted the bread for some thirty-five years. Hopefully, I'll get to taste it again. Fred shared the encouraging news recently that he still has the mixing bucket. I didn't ask, but suspect that it probably contains some remnants of the last loaf he made while in college. That next loaf he makes could be the best ever!

There was a dark side to Fred bread though. Fred consumed the bread by richly coating one piece with peanut butter, another with jelly, and placing them together to create peanut butter sandwiches. The problem was that Fred had an unbreakable habit of holding his sandwich perpendicular to the floor rather than horizontally, or parallel to the floor. If you are unable to visualize this, let me explain it another way. Fred carried his peanut butter and jelly sandwiches around the house in a way that permitted the peanut butter and jelly filling, mostly the jelly, to drip generously onto the floor. It then was mixed together with the normal ingredients to be found on the floor, such as dirt, dust and grime, as people walked through the house. The drippings took their place among the black polka-dotted pattern marking earlier baking efforts, making it difficult to tell the old from the new. The trick was never to go barefoot, and to try to avoid those spots less than a week old where the jelly might not yet have dried.

The Mystery of Dave's Sore Knees. The house was great for parties. Dave and I decided to organize one, and we took pains to have healthful beverages for our guests. We bought a large plastic hatbox to use for a bowl, and then made a punch with several gallons of different fruit juices, two gallons of vanilla ice cream (with natural vanilla flavor), and rum. I think we added some other odds and ends of different alcoholic beverages for complexity. I know grain alcohol was one. It was an impetuous little punch, much favored by our guests.

The ice cream coated the stomach, so that those of our guests who stuck with the punch really didn't do too badly. Dave and John, however, had a bottle of Yugoslavian plum brandy left by a friend on some prior visit. The two of them, inspired by some amorous pursuit of the moment, finished that as well. In the morning, or more precisely, the early afternoon, they attempted to rejoin the living. Both had hangovers of classic proportions, but Dave also reported a great pain in his knees. He hadn't a clue as to why, and indeed it remained a mystery until John regained the power of speech and explained that he had seen Dave crawling back and forth from his bedroom to the bathroom throughout the night.

Dave has turned out to be a fine lawyer, a loving father and a great friend. Dave, I don't know how you are going to command respect from your children once they see what you were like at their age. That is why I am making you this limited time offer. For a sum that is really modest given the extra burden of having special copies printed, I will prepare copies in which I substitute Fred for you in this section. Given the low demand expected for this version, I think a thousand dollars for each copy sounds reasonable. Let me know how many you want.

My Room (and Dave's before Me). I moved into this house to attend my first year of law school. As new kid on the block, I had to start in the room near the front of the house traditionally given to the person with least seniority. Dave had lived there once but had moved up in rank. It wasn't really a bedroom; it was an entry foyer, rendered unnecessary by some past change to the floor plan. It wasn't big enough for both a bed and a desk, both of which I needed. To make use of the space efficiently, I used a narrow piece of foam on the floor as my bed, and a small junior high-sized desk as my place of study.

The room would have been habitable but for one thing: it had two walls made of glass panes, many of which were cracked. I hadn't noticed this flaw in August when I moved in. It was impossible to ignore in January. I wore hooded sweatshirts and gloves when I studied or slept. Otherwise, I stayed out of my room when I could. My friends had great fun yelling at me for causing a draft whenever I opened my door to enter the rest of the house.

I moved out at the end of my first year because John was going on "Sea Semester," a supposed college course where you learned to sail by crossing the Atlantic. In addition, another inhabitant announced that he had befriended a professional stripper and that she was moving in. Strangely, my grades started improving immediately upon moving out of the house.

Dave Takes a Wife. Dave and I knew each other less well in our college years. I had moved to Washington, D.C., when I graduated law school, and he too found a job that brought him there. He called me asking for advice on lodging, and we agreed that he would stay with me while he looked for something more permanent. We looked for the loves of our lives when we were out, and fought a losing fight against the roaches in my apartment when we were in. The number of single women in Washington, D.C., and the number of cockroaches in my apartment were roughly the same, but we seemed to do better attracting the latter. At least I don't remember returning home and finding thirty or forty women in my apartment running for cover the minute I turned on the light.

I realize I am digressing from the story of friendship, but I feel an obligation to preserve what I learned in trying to fight large numbers of roaches at a time. War between cockroaches and humans in the future is inevitable, and it would be a tragedy if the lessons I learned in this early skirmish were lost. Remember this: evolution has made the roaches highly capable of sensing changes in light. Try and swat a roach, and it will detect the change in light caused by your hand and swiftly move out of the way.

Evolution did not prepare them for the tactical weapon I introduced into our fight: suction. They don't understand it. I could sneak the vacuum nozzle almost up to their ugly little heads without reaction. Then with a blast of suction they would be snatched out of the field of battle into a canister which contained, among other things, boric acid, a roach killer that was not harmful to humans. My vacuum became my weapon of choice. Roaches who dared show themselves became easy victims, so much so that I occasionally said things to others like "it is as easy as vacuuming roaches," forgetting that this would not be meaningful to them. I couldn't run the vacuum constantly, however, and I finally called it quits after waking up and finding squashed roaches in my bed.

Dave traded a life with me and the roaches for a more presentable apartment and the pursuit of Elsa. It seemed like a good trade at the time. Perhaps his first marriage was doomed when he asked me to be his best man, but I swear I had nothing to do with his second. Fortunately, his second wife, who was also his first, is married to her fourth husband if you count Dave twice, making it seem unlikely that he will marry her a third time. But I have learned never to rule anything out and to try instead to influence the odds by making fun of him about this. Perhaps if we had begun the jokes earlier, we could have spared him the second divorce. Dave, we're on the case, and we intend to play an active role in reviewing candidates for wife number three.

John Becomes a Success Thanks to Me. John never wanted to work for others and spent a number of years looking for opportunities to start his own operation, run it the way he thought it ought to be run, and make his fortune. That he accomplished this is a great tribute to him, and I disclaim any involvement in his current business of making some sort of over-priced test equipment for airplanes.

"But admit it, John; you wouldn't have made it without me! No? Excuse me, would you please return to the witness stand. I remind you, you're under oath." He is beginning to sweat a bit now, as he wonders what I am up to. "Isn't it true, Bowling Man, that you had many get-rich schemes you considered before you hit on the one that worked?"

Man oh man, the sweat is starting to bead on his lower lip and his forehead. He thinks he knows where I am going and turns to the judge and asks for a break. The judge, who will be taking a pleasant vacation at a place I own in the Virgin Islands, instructs John to quit sniveling, get back in the witness chair, and answer my questions or go to jail for contempt. John's lawyer tries to object, but the judge tells him to sit down and shut up, overruling this and any further objections that the lawyer might make that day, prospectively.

Time to move in for the kill. "Now, one of those schemes that you thought of pursuing was to make … (pregnant pause to build suspense towards a horrible, ego-crushing climax) … tugboat fenders!" The jury gasps, two women faint, and John hangs his head in shame before being escorted to a waiting van from Junior Achievement.

I swear that the part about tugboat fenders is true. Tugboats really do have fenders, and there is really a business, not a great business but a business, in making such things. Those of you who have jumped out of your chairs to go tear his test equipment out of your planes, sit down. Everyone can make a mistake. This was John's. Fortunately, John had the good sense to test the idea with others. I think the sound of my laughter, while perhaps not welcome at the time, played some small part in his decision to preserve his capital for a better opportunity. If not for me, he would probably stink of fish, be relatively poor, and be driving a rusted out pick-up rather than the sleek new car that he bought so he could drive us around on our last trip. I almost hate to mention it, but John did eventually hit on something that seemed to work, and he built a company that became so wildly successful that when he decided to sell, he had more offers to buy his company than the combined number of offers I have received in my lifetime to buy every house I have lived in, added to the offers to buy every car I have owned.

Our Vacations. The four of us stayed in loose touch for a number of years. Then, about fifteen years ago, John suggested the four of us get together for a short vacation. No one can quite remember everything we've done, but we seem to meet roughly every one or two years, going to Banff, Zion, Yellowstone, Whistler, the White Mountains in New Hampshire, Napa and other such places. These are special times. There is nothing that can compare to friendships that have endured. We totally accept and support each other. We know the failures, the strengths and weaknesses of each other, and have shared in the sorrows and joys almost as if we were old married people. Invariably, people who meet us and learn of the friendship's history look at us wistfully and express the wish that they had something similar.

These trips have been so wonderful that I really didn't think that they could get better. It was my illness that proved me wrong. I am writing this in my hotel room in San Francisco at the end of this year's trip. I have had Parkinson's disease for a number of years, but had always been able to suppress the symptoms with medication so that it wouldn't interfere with our activities. Recently, the symptoms have been progressing rapidly and are now beyond the reach of available medications. This year, I would fidget and writhe in restaurants, unable to sit still. I also suffered constant back pain due to muscle spasms. For the first time, I was unable to participate in the physical activity that was planned, in this case a modest hike. But perhaps my biggest impact on the trip was my changed behavior, exhibiting an almost manic obsession with having fun now that could at times cause me to act as if I were out of control.

They could have been annoyed. They had a right to be, because their time is precious and I was acting in ways that made it less fun for them. As I prepare to tell you what you already have guessed, my eyes are becoming misty all over again. My friends put aside what they may have wanted to do, and instead devoted themselves to making the trip fun for me. They looked out for me, put their arms around my shoulders and hugged me. I feel truly loved, and I count myself lucky to have friends like this. I don't know if I'll ever be able to make another one of these trips. Even if I do, I can't imagine this trip ever being equaled. I have been to the mountaintop!

I've had a fascinating life, and I hope to have other wonderful experiences. Still, this is a fitting occasion to say thanks to the best friends a man could have. John, David and Fred, thank you from the bottom of my heart. The last revelation I will make about you is that you are a bunch of softies, who do a poor job of hiding your feelings. Stay that way.

They have. When I had my brain surgery, not one but all three came to see me through my convalescence. They were somewhat surprised that the day after surgery I was challenging them to games of ping pong. They were very surprised that I won consistently. No, they didn't allow me to beat them. You don't know these guys.

I did not totally waste the rest of my educational years. After my first year of undergraduate work, I decided to drop out of school and travel the world. I started off those travels by spending about six months on a kibbutz in Israel. You couldn't beat it—free room and board and seven dollars a month in pay! I learned more during that year than any of the years I spent obtaining my undergraduate degree. I even made some progress with women, which will cost you a lot more than the price of this book to hear about.

I will share one experience even at the expense of personal reputation, because it fits with a life-long tendency, wherever I am, to have experiences slightly off center. I don't go looking for these things; they just seem to happen. While I was on the kibbutz, the man who was responsible for their program of artificial insemination of the large chicken population went into the army, as most Israeli males do for some period of each year. This is not a political comment on the situation in the Middle East, but merely to explain why they needed to fill a void that his reserve duty created.

I should have been more suspicious when they not only looked to replace him with people who had never worked on a farm before, such as myself, but also bribed us with promises that when we got really good at doing it, we would be able to get the work done in less than two hours and have the rest of the day free! Enticed by the prospect of having more time to spend chasing a French girl with whom I was infatuated, I volunteered.

The idea behind artificial insemination is to bring fertilization rates up. Apparently, roosters are no different in some ways than men. They prefer some chicks over others, and many of the chickens are neglected, even though they have nice personalities and would make fine mothers. One way of looking at what we did was that we were ensuring that every chicken was treated the same, no matter her looks. Another way was that we were indeed collecting semen from roosters who weren't very happy about it, and then using soft tipped hypodermic needles to deposit what we collected into more chickens held upside down than you can imagine. I still bear the scars, physical and emotional, from this job. As for the French girl, she threw me over anyway.

It could have been worse. When the true expert at this job came back, he started looking for volunteers to help him do similar work with cattle. One look at the bull and I decided to go work in the bakery.

PART V:

The Years in the District of Columbia: Marriage and Fatherhood

I told my son that he owes his life to an ugly suit I bought in Filene's basement and used for job interviews. He humored me with a small laugh, but it is true. I had strong law school credentials. My grades picked up the last two years allowing me to graduate near the top of my class, and I did well in activities like moot court (where my partner and I won the school competition). Still, I couldn't land a job. I had plenty of interviews, but kept being passed over in favor of others who, at least on paper, had lesser credentials.

Did I mention the suit? I had purchased it at Filene's basement, a landmark of Boston shopping. It was the last stop for garments. Here they were sold without dignity to shoppers who were willing to buy and wear clothing that had been passed up, generally with good reason, by every one of the hundreds of customers who had looked at them earlier in their history.

The suit I picked out, a loud grey and red plaid three-piece mistake by Yves St. Laurent, continued a pattern of dressing inappropriately for events of great importance to me. It is possible that I was doing this deliberately for some twisted psychological reason, but more likely it was because I had terrible taste and was oblivious to the effect my clothes had on others. The suit did not equal the bell-bottom pants in pure repulsive effect, but when you added to the suit a tie that did not match (as I did), the cumulative effect was close.

Perhaps I am wrong to blame my lack of success on my clothing rather than taking responsibility for falling short in other areas. Certainly the law school I went to—Boston University—did not have the reputation of some others, so job offers had to be earned by individual achievement rather than the aura of the school I attended. Nor was I the perfect candidate. It seems too coincidental, however, that the one offer I did receive resulted from an informal interview where I did *not* wear the suit. It was a small law firm in Washington, D.C., now known as Cole, Raywid & Braverman. The pay was substantially less than offered by the larger firms. Truthfully, I probably wouldn't have even interviewed there had I received an early lucrative job offer from one of the larger firms.

Working there turned out to be an incredibly lucky break, not just for my son, who was born because of it, but also for me. I had incredible fun, and the experiences I had at the beginning of my career were beyond anything I would have experienced at the larger firms. While large-firm associates were practicing for the big time doing document reviews, writing memos and taking depositions under the watchful eyes of more senior attorneys, I was plunged into the big time, sink or swim. In my first year, I wrote a brief for the United States Supreme Court on behalf of the United States Senate and Senator Proxmire, and helped try an antitrust case against AT&T in Rapid City, South Dakota. We lost both. The following year I asked to argue the appeal of the AT&T antitrust case in lieu of my friend and mentor, Alan Raywid. Despite it being the firm's most significant case, he convinced his partners to let me do it. We won a 3-0 reversal in the Court of Appeals. I didn't stop celebrating for months!

Janis and I met because I worked at the firm, and I worked at the firm because of the suit. She lived next to an associate at the firm, and when she decided to have a leap year party, she asked him to invite some unattached attorneys from the office to attend. I went because he had described his neighbor as a very pretty lady, also unattached. It wasn't set up as a blind date for the two of us, but it might as well have been. We hit it off and spent most of the party in each other's company.

Janis and I traveled in such different circles that I am reasonably certain that had I not met her at that party, we would not have met. Without going to the firm, I wouldn't have been at the party. Without the suit... You get the picture.

Meeting at the party was a first step, but it took other interventions by fate to cause my son's birth. This requires a slight digression from the previous digression to explain.

I had moved from the roach motel and joined my old friend Dave and another buddy of his in a group house up near Livingston Circle. We were three, the house had four bedrooms, and the addition of another tenant would cut our rent. We placed an advertisement in the paper, and the first person to answer was Angie, an effervescent black woman who we all liked immediately. She did not seem deterred at the prospect of living with us, so who were we to complain?

All went well until the night of Janis' party. It was extraordinarily cold, and on my way home my car stalled and wouldn't restart. I left it parked on Capitol Hill where it had died and took a bus home. Angie offered to drive me to it the next morning. The cold had also brought snow and ice to the road, and Angie lost control of her car after we had driven one block. It slammed into the curb, bending one of the axles. Though I offered to pay half of the deductible because she had been doing me a favor, I thought she should also assume some responsibility for talking with her hands, touching the wheel only between gestures, while driving too fast on a sheet of ice. In the days and weeks that followed, I was greeted each day with the auto repair report followed by repeats of the daytime soap, *You Ruined My Life, You Car Killer*, followed by nightly ambushes when, no matter how late I arrived, I was presented with angry remonstrations at my indifference to her vehicular tragedy.

What had been a pleasant house became a place to avoid. I decided to move out. Janis too needed to move because her lease was up. She proposed that we find a place and live together. It took me about five seconds to agree—we were in the bloom of a new romance, and I was swept away with the utter romance of setting up house with her.

I look at pictures of the two of us taken at the time and know from the way we looked at each other that we were indeed in love. We were married a year later, and our son Hank was born a couple of years after that. It's difficult to look back with any sort of objectivity and figure out why it didn't last. There is probably no single truth.

This being my book, however, I am the one who gets to guess. It was all her fault. I was a saint. That may be too simplistic for those who require understanding of the deep psychological underpinnings of marital discord rather than accepting as I have that it is the natural order of things. For them, I offer the following. Janis was quick to embrace new things, taking them on with unbounded exuberance, but the enthusiasm would run its course, sometimes quickly, and she would be ready to move on. I am much slower to embrace new things, but when I do, my interest in them lasts longer than hers. Put us together and we were almost always out of sync—she would become enthusiastic about something in which I would have little interest. Then, about the time she was becoming bored with it and was ready to move on, I would pick up the banner, become its biggest fan, and stick with it for a long, long time.

For those of you who find that explanation a bunch of hooey, please feel free to revert to the equally good explanation that preceded it. It was all her fault; I was a saint. What is truly amazing is that my second marriage seems to be in trouble for the exact same reason. Now what are the odds against that?

I left the small firm after three years when I disappointed them by asking for more money and they disappointed me by saying no. I moved to a larger firm, now called Dickstein, Shapiro, Morin & O'Shinsky. It was located at 21st and L. Janis and I moved to a condo at 22nd and P. The distance between the two was about five blocks. I sold my car and walked to work. Life was good, but it had a few bugs that needed working out.

I was still doing litigation and worked for a superb litigator who prided himself on being a tyrant. He had a lot for which he could be proud. I worked like a dog and hardly saw my son for the first six months of his life. I learned a lot in the three years I was there, about both law and my own views on what is important in life.

I remember working on an antitrust case which took me to warehouses around the country looking for documents. I had just finished a long day in Atlanta going through boxes of papers that hadn't seen the light of day for years, and had come back to my motel room to wash the dust from my body, have a quick bite to eat and go to bed. My message light was on. The tyrant had called. He wanted me to fly up that night to meet with him at the firm's NYC apartment. Thinking something urgent must have happened, I quickly packed and caught the last flight to New York. Once there I raced to the apartment trying to think what made it so necessary that I get there that evening.

He let me in, dressed in an undershirt and boxers. He asked how my day had been, and then, patting his ample belly, asked me to tell him *whether I thought he looked fat*! I don't remember my answer. What I do remember was that after I said whatever I said, he yawned and said he was going to bed. That was it. I slept on the sofa and added this to my store of reasons to begin looking for another job.

I answered a blind ad in the Wall Street Journal placed by AT&T. AT&T offered me more money than I had been making for work I was certain would be less demanding. I took the job. I would get to see my son more, and make more money for working fewer hours.

There was another reason that we wanted to move. Our condo was adjacent in the back to a gay bar that had outdoor fashion shows for its guests that began at 11:00 p.m. The bar did not want to move the entertainment inside because they drew a larger crowd outdoors. I was not then the nocturnal creature I have become; my wife and son weren't even close. It is a question of one's perspective as to who was the nuisance, but legally I believe we were in the right and they were in the wrong.

Had they been willing to discuss the matter we probably would have compromised in some manner. They offered no accommodation, however, so we challenged their license. In doing so, I learned two things: first, there are no legal bars in Washington, D.C., and second, it doesn't really matter.

The ordinances in Washington, D.C., required then, and as far as I know still require, that every "restaurant" make more than half its revenues from the sale of food. Every bar I went to in the six years I lived there served hamburgers or some other light fare, but I honestly don't think a single establishment with which I was familiar, which was a respectable number, met that standard. If my expenditures on food and alcohol in such places were at all typical, they wouldn't even have come close. It was the law, however, and a solution needed to be found so that the Alcoholic Beverage Control ("ABC") Board didn't have to enforce it.

For those of you unfamiliar with D.C. politics, I assure you that the Board looked at the challenge to the license for a popular gay bar brought by a young white professional with justifiable horror. They did what any self-perpetuating group of corruptible bureaucrats would do—they made a "surprise" inspection of the place around midnight, found it quiet except for the usual restaurant-type noise of patrons eating their dinners, and then told us to work something out because they had no intention of ruling on this case. Fifteen minutes before the inspection, and fifteen minutes after, the bar was its usual, noisy self. I love surprises.

We settled. They agreed to quiet down around midnight on weekends and 11 pm on weekdays. These were not bad terms, but the times were still a bit late for a four-month-old baby. It gave additional reason to move. A marvelous feature about AT&T's offer to me was that they would buy the condo if we were unable to sell it. We had overpaid for it in the first place, and they offered more than we had paid, and far more than we would have been able to get for it.

This made me grateful that I was going to work for the world's most powerful corporation. It would be fun to have that kind of muscle on your side. What could go wrong?

PART VI:

A Personal, Abbreviated Eulogy to AT&T

I spent slightly more than two decades working for AT&T. I joined the company as a junior lawyer in 1983, and worked my way up the ranks before retiring as a Vice President in August, 2004. It was purely coincidental, but during the same twenty-one years, AT&T went from being the most powerful company in the world to a company barely keeping its head above water. It worked its way down as I worked my way up. It was not my fault.

At its peak, AT&T sat atop an incredibly powerful group of companies that dominated everything they touched. Its local companies, the Bell Operating Companies, were legal monopolies which served nearly every desirable market in the country. The less populated areas were served by some 1600 smaller independent companies that existed at AT&T's sufferance. Its research arm, Bell Laboratories, attracted the finest minds in the world. Bell Labs invented most of the technologies now used in telecommunications, including cellular technology, fiber optics, the laser, and digital radio. AT&T scientists discovered the "Big Bang," tracing the background noise in radio transmissions to the explosion billions of years ago that marked the creation of the universe, and they invented the transistor, hailed as the most important invention of the twentieth century, as a replacement for vacuum tubes then used in communications equipment. The equipment itself was made by Western Electric, fully owned by AT&T, and the largest manufacturer of telecom equipment in the world.

At the time of its demise, AT&T had fallen so low that its death was barely considered newsworthy and was not reported in many papers. It had become a shadow of its former self, with shrinking revenues forcing lay-off after lay-off until finally it was purchased in 2005 by one of the companies it had spun off in the 1980s. The popular wisdom is that it was a victim of its own poor management. The popular wisdom is wrong. Ma Bell, as the company was known, was killed by the only one who could have done it—Uncle Sam. Accepting every allegation of mismanagement at face value, the fact remains that the company's missteps, though costing it billions, were a nit compared to the things done to it by government.

I have struggled *without success* to find a succinct way to tell what happened. Told *un*succinctly, the story meanders through arcane regulatory rules, known to cause brain damage to those laboratory rats who tried to understand their logic, and is about as enjoyable as watching footage of the Hindenburg disaster over and over. Those of my test readers who did not throw themselves off cliffs begged to escape this part, making me think it still needed a tweak or two.

I surrendered to the inevitable and decided that this was not the time or the place to tell the full AT&T story. Perhaps some day I will write an account of what really happened. For now, with the aid of this lengthy introduction and a few gross over-simplifications, I have reduced the saga to little more than a page or two.

In the late 1940s, AT&T scientists invented the transistor, a world-changing discovery. It revealed the invention to the public in the early 1950s. A thankful government brought an antitrust action against the company, fearing that the company might extend its power into the young world of computers. The decree settling the lawsuit prohibited the company from entering the computer business, made it divest its international operations, and required the company to license all of its then or future patents to any who wanted to use them.

In the 1980s the government sued again and broke up the company into local and long distance companies. Before the break-up, AT&T had kept local rates low by a complex set of internal cross subsidies, essentially using long distance profits to make local service affordable. The government, not wanting the break-up of the company to be perceived as causing increases in local rates, forced the now separate long distance companies to continue paying subsidies to the local companies.

Between 1984 and the time it was acquired, AT&T paid the local companies more than a *quarter trillion* dollars in such subsidies. There is no inherent logic to the charges other than historical Bell System practice. The payments placed AT&T at an intolerable competitive disadvantage, not to mention made the company a quarter trillion dollars poorer. When the local companies were authorized to enter long distance and began competing with AT&T, the company could no longer survive. The fat lady sang her song, and that was that.

The government recently has permitted the recombination of the local and long distance companies, forming two companies, one with headquarters in Texas, and one headquartered in New York. Western Electric (renamed Lucent somewhere along the way) has been acquired by Alcatel, meaning that Bell Laboratories and the last U.S. manufacturer of much of the equipment that goes into telephone networks is now owned by the French. Don't get me wrong. I think the French make wonderful wine and cheese. But tell the truth: When was the last time you used the words "French" and "technology" in the same sentence?

(In my official capacity as this book's author, I want you to know that I deplore insults against entire countries. "I like the French people. I really do." And you may quote me on that.)

I fought in the wars to preserve AT&T and lost. It hurt. And I loved the Red Sox for years too, and gave up on them after decades of frustration only to see them win it all the next year. That really hurt. I voted against George Bush twice. That one is killing me. You see why I refuse to give in to disease? The law of averages requires that I win something soon, or the universe will spin madly out of control. And, my dear universe, if you think for one minute that I am going to count that free cookbook I won in the supermarket scratch-off game but didn't even pick up, you've got another thought coming. I'm talking a meaningful win here, not some unimportant little triumph. Do you really want to spin out of control with the other parallel universes watching?

PART VII:

Diogenes Steals My Television, and Other Misadventures in the World of Business

I have always liked the Greek myth about Diogenes, who carried around a lantern looking for an honest man. I was surprised, however, when a man matching his description, lantern and all, knocked on my door last month and identified himself as the very Diogenes of whom the stories were written. Suspecting a scam, I asked to see some identification, and was not surprised when he failed to produce any. I told him to take a hike, but he looked so wounded that I relented and let him come in. I warmed up some food left over from dinner for him and brought him a blanket so that he could sleep on the sofa. He looked tired and grateful. The next morning he was gone, as was my stereo and television. In its place were his lantern and a note that read: "Please feel free to continue the quest. I give up. Thanks for the hospitality." It was signed "Diogenes."

This cynical little fable is good training for those who would enter the world of business. I do not know whether it was always so, but honesty in this world today is a rare commodity. Try to maintain high ethical standards and you are considered naïve.

The interludes below cover a variety of things with one common theme—they are things which we accept that we should not. Forgive me while I get back on my soap box and at least poke some fun at those who do these things.

Tenth Interlude:

Mail-in Rebates—A Case for a Small Holy War

Jihad! As one generally among the target class addressed by that word, I can feel its power and would love to have such passion on my side. It is a tremendous force we Westerners could really use. I don't know if we may use it for our purposes, or whether it can only be used where the core tenets of religion are involved. I can see the danger in over-utilization. One can't use it for just anything and still have people ready to blow themselves and others up when they hear the word. A jihad against the Nets moving to Long Island, as much as I'd like it, would not feel right.

We Westerners need something that would strike fear in the hearts of our targets. Crusade! That doesn't really do it. Banzai! It's good but it's not ours. We really don't have anything suitable. Our language ("Remember the Maine" or Remember the Alamo" or "Remember Pearl Harbor") reflects a national reluctance to throw the first punch. We just don't have a ready store of battle cries that we can hurl at our enemies, scaring them into submission. The closest example comes from the movies, not real life, and was a question rather than a statement. "Do you feel lucky, punk?"

We will have to launch a holy war first, and come up with a suitable battle cry later. Our first target: companies that use mail-in rebates to lie to, torment and overcharge you. We suffer quietly because we wonder whether we're the only ones who can't seem to perform the tasks that the companies offering the rebates assign to us. You're not alone!

What is so bad about requiring people who want the advertised rebate to send in a form?

Let's start with a question: why do companies use rebate programs? Wouldn't it be simpler just to reduce the price? Sure. It costs the company less too. Rebate programs are expensive. One needs employees to perform the otherwise unnecessary jobs the rebate program requires—collecting and processing the rebate forms, for example. Why then do companies incur the extra expense? They spend the money for rebate programs because they save more money avoiding the payment of discounts to their customers than they spend on the program itself. Simply said, they will throw one dollar in the garbage to avoid giving you the two dollars they led you to believe you would get back as a rebate.

Think about that. The companies advertise the price after rebate, and then create obstacle courses to prevent their customers from gaining the benefit described. They do more than count on customers being lazy; they take affirmative steps to make it difficult for customers to get the advertised prices.

Wouldn't it be nice if you could easily find the rebate form? They're generally available at a web site patterned after *Where's Waldo*. The key to obtaining the right rebate form is there somewhere if you could just find it. What about calling them up? "Hello. This is John. How may I assist you? Send you forms? I'm sorry, there is a mail strike here in Bombay." More recently, the people in the call centers simply say they are "unauthorized" to provide such forms and advise you to go back to the web site. Even if you get the form, don't think you're done. You're not.

I recently acquired a "free cell phone" after rebate in exchange for signing up with my wireless service provider for another two years. A very courteous salesperson actually handed me a rebate form. I looked at it when I got home and discovered the type was too small for me to read. I tried various techniques—holding the form up to a light, or tilting my glasses to get extra magnification—just to read it. I finally was able to read enough words to understand that I had to write a fifteen digit number in little boxes. The number was not on any of the documentation or sales receipts. Those numbers could have verified the sale, but those weren't the ones they wanted.

The number they required could be found by disassembling the phone, removing the battery, and looking on the internal housing on the phone. Of course, why didn't I think of that in the first place? I tried my best to read it, but in the end I had to guess at a few digits. Three months later, I received a letter denying the rebate. I had guessed incorrectly. They offered me another chance if I had another original receipt (which I didn't). In all, I have purchased three phones over the last year for members of my family. Each had a rebate, but I've yet to be able to turn any into cash.

The wireless guys are amateurs compared to McAfee. At the time I wrote this, McAfee was running a rebate program that won the award for the nastiest rebate program I have encountered. My wireless provider had merely made it difficult to obtain the offered rebate; McAfee made it impossible.

McAfee used a very effective tactic to get people to purchase continuing software updates, bombarding your computer constantly with pop-up messages warning you of trouble unless you renewed your service. I couldn't figure out how to end the pop-up bombardment so, in frustration, I bought the update. Cost was listed at $48, after mail-in rebate. What you discovered after your purchase was that to qualify for the rebate, you had to have the receipt and original box and packaging, not from what you just bought, but from the original McAfee software that may have been purchased years earlier! Moreover, if your computer came with the original McAfee software already installed, you were not eligible for the rebate! In other words, many if not most people are ineligible for the rebate when they make the purchase, and there's not a thing they can do about it unless they can change the past.

This kind of dishonesty should not become part of accepted commercial practice. Here are some ways we can stop it!

Next time you're tempted to buy something because an applicable rebate makes the price seem attractive, send a letter to the President of the company instead, letting him know that you didn't buy the product because of the company's use of mail-in-rebates. The following could serve as a model: "Dear Mr. _____, I have decided not to buy your products because of your use of mail-in rebates. Why are you offering a rebate and then making it difficult to obtain? Didn't you have parents who taught you right from wrong, or are you doing this in the hope that they don't find out? It might be useful if you copy them on your response, because I sent them a copy of this letter."

Seriously, perhaps we should create some system to have the actions of the top corporate executives reviewed by their mothers. Today, there is no accountability on senior executives so long as they make the numbers and aren't caught breaking the law. They act on behalf of their shareholders and under the supervision of their Boards. I was a corporate lawyer for twenty-one years, the last ten at senior levels within one of the best companies in the country. I had many friends who worked at other companies, also at senior positions. The notion that the company leadership must answer to either board or shareholders in any meaningful way is a nice idea, but it isn't really accurate.

Few if any board members understand what goes on at this level in the companies on whose boards they sit. In fact many of them are selected (nominations are normally made by company management) because they are already friendly to management, or are not overly inquisitive individuals. Corporate CEOs wouldn't try half the nonsense on their mothers that they now routinely convince their boards to accept.

The shareholders are even less of a concern. Most don't have a clue what goes on in the company they "own," and there is no way for a small shareholder to call a CEO to task. In contrast, mothers have a way of cutting through the window dressing and getting to the point. I would love just once to hear something like, "Johnny, I don't care who started it. I want you to give him back his money and stop trying to overcharge everybody for your product, or you'll spend the rest of the night in your room."

Second, the Federal Trade Commission has jurisdiction over false advertising and has stringent rules regarding the misuse of the word "free" as in my "free" cell phones. Hello! Is there anyone home? Wake up! We're talking slam dunk here.

Third, the states have escheat laws on the books providing that unclaimed property escheats to (or becomes the property of) the state. Yes, these laws are antiquated. That hasn't stopped the states from enforcing them in other circumstances. Why not here? It seems reasonable to assert that the discount offered in a rebate coupon is an item of property owned by the customer, not the vendor, and if the customer fails to claim it, then it belongs to the state. If your current statute doesn't support this position, that's not a permanent problem. Change the statute!

This will be fun! While we are at it, I will keep working on our battle cry. It's not that I dislike the "do you feel lucky, punk?" question posed by Dirty Harry. It's just that this threat lacks the quick hitting punch of the one-word threats used by others. Hopefully, Mr. Eastwood will read this and make another movie or two in which he can supply a more succinct epithet to hurl at those he is about to shoot. I want to get these guys, not talk them to death.

The funeral industry would not be my favorite, even if those in it were very ethical. I have had too much experience with it in recent years. My mother-in-law died early in 2004; my own mother passed away towards the end of the same year. As a result I got to see the industry up close and personal. While some of the individuals working in the industry seem very nice and caring, these commendable traits do not seem to prevent them from capitalizing on the family's grief in order to sell to the family very expensive, and totally pointless items. Maybe they aren't as nice as they seem...

ELEVENTH INTERLUDE:
WOULD YOU LIKE CREMAINS WITH YOUR COFFIN?

Surely you have heard of "cremains." They are the human remains resulting from cremation. The word was given us by the funeral industry and is used by practitioners with great solemnity. "And how shall we be handling the cremains? We have a number of tasteful urns starting at one thousand dollars. Or, if you prefer to spend less, we carry a line of clay pots from China. Of course they disintegrate more rapidly than porcelain, and there is a risk to the 'cremains.'"

Why do we tolerate such an industry? Death should be commemorated so that the dead can get on with their death, and the living can get on with their lives. Instead it has become yet another business opportunity where the living are shamed into spending silly amounts of money to prove their grief. The dead don't care much how they look, what kind of coffin they're in, etc. But small fortunes nonetheless are expended making certain they look and have the best because the living are made to think that others will think less of them if they spend too little.

There are some things I abhor but that I accept. Draining the blood from a dead person and then painting his face so that he "looks alive" and can be viewed one last time makes me cringe. To others it seems to be part of closure. But there are other things that just don't make any sense. Cremation, which could be a sensible way of postponing the day when every square foot of the earth has been turned into a cemetery, has become a completely silly and redundant process where we first dispose of the body and then act as if we haven't.

What is the point of cremating the body if we still bury it? We are using more and more land as final resting places for the dead. What exactly are we burying after the body is cremated? Trick question. Those who answered "the dead guy" must take their seats. It's the cremains, and supposedly the ashes from that expensive coffin you bought, forever mixed together.

When you start the process of selecting your very special cremation, the first stop on your shopping tour is to view the variety of coffins to hold the body when it is cremated. Whatever you choose will be turned to dust in a few brief minutes' exposure to thousand degree temperatures. I don't mean to be flip, but buying a very expensive casket to burn is a little like buying a new Porsche and taking it to a demolition derby.

Why does the grieving family spend tens of thousands of dollars on a beautiful, handcrafted masterpiece of a coffin, only to incinerate it with their loved one? As was patiently explained to us, New Jersey law, which applied to my mother-in-law's body, prohibited cremation without using some kind of container, at least a cardboard coffin. (Somehow, I don't think the legislature thought that up on its own.) It must be very good cardboard because it costs more than four hundred dollars. But it pales in comparison to the top line caskets that can cost thousands.

Do you really believe that they burn those beautiful coffins? I suspect not. Generally, no one attends this particular part of the process.

Perhaps there is an "underground railroad" for coffins where they are spirited out of one state and reach safety in another where they can be sold once again. I hope no one is incensed. The last thing in the world we need to see is a crackdown on the funeral industry that results in them burning these works of art. What would that accomplish other than increased waste? What we need to do is address the real problem—the decedent's family's decision to pick that expensive coffin in the first place. Why do they do it?

Picture yourself in the funeral home. All there look sad, the funeral director most of all. Many of the family members are feeling some measure of guilt for something they did or didn't do to or for the decedent prior to his death. The family is made to feel that it could be a tremendous embarrassment if they picked a "cheap" cardboard coffin. "Yes, we had mother cremated in a very tasteful cardboard container. You should have seen it; it was beautiful." Your choice, ma'am, cardboard or mahogany? Now what do you think?

Let's do a final total here on what happened to cremation as a potentially efficient procedure. We have two containers for the body—the one in which the body is burned and the one in which the ashes are buried. A traditional funeral would use only one. We have two expensive events—the cremation and the internment of the "cremains." Again, we are one up on tradition. No land use benefits because we still use the land. What could have been a more efficient process has been headed off at the pass and turned into one that is more expensive at every turn.

Or should I say "...at every urn." This pun is an excuse to mention a bit of personal history. Following my mother-in-law's death, we looked at the urns in the funeral parlor but found none that we liked. Prices exceeded a thousand dollars, on average. As luck would have it we received a Fortunoff advertisement in the mail. On a whim I looked through it quickly and found several enameled urns, more beautiful than any we'd seen, and costing less than two hundred dollars. We received a number of compliments.

I don't believe in presenting problems without at least offering solutions. Let's tackle it piece by piece.

When someone dies, the family does not know what to do. They are now in charge of a body. The hospital staff is helpful, and asks, "And what will you be doing with the body?" They then reassure the panicked family. No need to worry. "Call a funeral director; they'll know what to do." In truth funeral directors do perform services, coordinating everything and arranging for the death certificate. But there is a temptation to which they too often succumb. In their trust is a family that is vulnerable, feeling dependent on them for guidance, and who really doesn't know how much to spend. It's like chum in the water.

The family's situation bears similarities to the situation of someone who has been arrested; they are isolated in an environment they don't understand, susceptible to intimidation, and badly in need of information. So why not treat the family as well as we do someone we think may have just committed a heinous crime?

As you may recall, prior to Miranda, police on some occasions were using the isolation following arrest to "extract" confessions. After waiting decades for elected officials to do something, the Supreme Court under Chief Justice Earl Warren stepped in and required—in the absence of some other solution—the reading of the arrested person's rights—the "Miranda warning"—to those arrested. It destroyed the isolation and required that they be given certain information to make it more difficult to lead them astray. Something similar would work here.

Imagine the following: When the family first met with the funeral director, they would be handed a card explaining their rights. They would be asked to sign a receipt that they had received it. Without a signed receipt, the funeral director's bill would not have to be paid. Here is a first draft of what the card would say:

Your Rights as a Survivor

1. We are sorry for your loss. Spending a lot of money on the dead does not make them any happier. They are dead, or should be, before you bury them.

2. We know the funeral director looks sad. He is not sad because of your loss. If anything, he is sad because more of your family didn't die at the same time. It would take more money than you have to make him happy.

3. You will be shown a lot of very expensive coffins, urns, flower arrangements, etc., and we know you want to show your respect for the dead. If you have unlimited amounts of money, please get the best of everything. If you do not, remember the living. People will understand if you decide to use your money to put your kids through college rather than incinerating your lost family member in an expensive casket. If they don't understand that, they are probably funeral directors.

4. Information on what funerals should cost and competitive alternatives in your area may be obtained from the Funeral Consumers Alliance at www.funerals.org.

Have a nice day.

Next is the question of what regulation we should impose to ensure the funeral industry deals with the grieving family in an honest way. Here's where I agree with my Republican friends. Other than the notice and labeling provisions, I vote for no regulation. In fact let's completely unshackle the industry.

The first part of my proposed legislation would read: "Notwithstanding anything in your contract to the contrary, a funeral home may cremate the deceased in anything they want to, and may save for future use any coffin sold, even if they promised to incinerate the deceased in it." If such a law existed, and the families were made aware of it, how many would still pay for that expensive coffin? Apply the same tactics to the urns and so forth. Much of the pressure to spend the big bucks would dissipate.

There is also the problem of the family worrying about what people would think. This is where labeling could work miracles. To counteract the high pressure sales tactics based on "what people will think," the legislation would mandate uniform labeling across the industry: Caskets or urns up to a total of $500 would be labeled "standard," $500 to $1000 would be "deluxe," $1000 to $2000 would be labeled "ostentatious," and above $2000 the label would be "unbelievably idiotic." The newness of this tactic will cause some of you to laugh and conclude I don't really mean it. But I do. The funeral industry has been using the "what will people think" tactic to induce billions in wasteful spending that many could ill afford. Let's reverse the tables. "Yes, I believe we'd like to have an unbelievably idiotic funeral, and we'll take that ostentatious coffin even though you may keep the money and never use it." Granted some people will spend the money, but not too many.

Before I leave this topic, I want to assure those who work in this industry that I know that many of them are nice people and that I have nothing personal against them. It is possible to be nice and still be a bloodsucker by profession. I know; I was a lawyer. So stop being so defensive and fix some of this stuff. You're going to find it harder to sell "unbelievably idiotic" funerals anyway.

One final thought. My own mother died recently. She left her body to science. The university that agreed to take her body sent very kind and caring people who arrived promptly after we called them the night she died. They were courteous yet extremely efficient and took her body away. That was it. Cost to the family: nothing. Not a brass farthing.

A few days later we had a lovely and much less stressful service. No one had to worry about the care and handling of her body, and I believe it contributed to the wonderful atmosphere at the service. There was no need to hang on to her corpse in order to remember her. It was so like her, taking advantage of this last opportunity to help others. Maybe at some point there will be a surplus of bodies that people wish to donate. But for now, this is an opportunity to do humanity a favor and save a lot of money at the same time. It doesn't get any better than that, at least with funerals.

PART VIII:

THE PURSUIT OF LOVE

The richness of life comes not only from work but also play and the pursuit of romance. I have always found work easy in comparison. Judging by the people I know well enough to discuss these sorts of things, others share this problem.

I do not intend an exhaustive treatment of my marriage to Mary. It is a history that is still being written in real life, and I do not wish this memoir to outpace or affect our actual lives. I can always leave the threat hanging in the air of coming back to this subject in the future, just as I did with the more detailed history of AT&T. There is little harm, I hope, in offering a few snippets of our early life together.

We met playing softball together on an intramural team at AT&T. Actually, I remember my first romantic thought was triggered when I was coaching first base and she was thrown out on a ground ball. I believe I gave her a sympathetic hug, which seemed the natural extension of my coaching responsibilities. I was dating someone else at the time, however, and I did not ask Mary out until that had run its course.

In many ways, Mary was the opposite of my first wife. I don't remember if I consciously thought, "I tried an art student and it didn't work; why don't I try an engineer?" If I had, it certainly would have fit the women involved. Mary had an engineering degree, and when we met she was a single mother working during the day and beginning to go to school at night to get her MBA. She had tremendous energy, something I attributed solely to her personality and only later connected to what she suffered from, bipolar disorder. She was an over-achiever against all odds. A divorced mother at twenty, she started in a trailer park in Iowa, and worked while she put herself through college, getting her undergraduate degree at the University of Iowa. She started her career at a large Western Electric facility in the Midwest before transferring to Western's headquarters location in New Jersey where we met. I have met few people in my life who could have done what she did.

We had a low-key wedding. It was just the two of us. We were married in Bermuda in the justice of the peace's office in a trip that combined wedding and honeymoon. Our wedding photo was taken against a wall painted to look like an island scene, snapped with a small pocket camera by a clerk we borrowed for the task. I don't believe either of us missed the absence of pomp and circumstance, and I likewise don't attribute our current issues to the absence of a big, formal wedding. We have attended such affairs for others who married after us, and split before us. In my view, such send-offs to married life do little to add to the sense of commitment of those involved. Of course, if you changed a thing or two....

TWELFTH INTERLUDE:
A MODEST PROPOSAL TO SAVE MARRIAGES AND STIMULATE THE ECONOMY

This whole thing started when a good friend of mine informed us that he and his lovely bride of not quite two years had decided to separate. The first thought that occurred to me, being as shallow as I am, was that this seemed to be somewhat of a short run given the cost of the event that had united them. I'm not talking about unusual extravagance: a rented hall, catered dining, flowers, booze, music, fancy clothes, gifts, photographers, limos, a love nest for the evening and more. It mounts up. I guessed the tally would hit ten thousand dollars, but my cost estimate may suffer from the same lack of imagination that I had when my wife proposed that we do a little landscaping.

I'm not a fanatic who believes that you should honor your vows and not part till death. I've proven that. There does come a time where parting is more bliss than sweet sorrow. Yet shouldn't we also think about those who paid for the wedding? Isn't it a little unseemly if the marriage ends while they are still paying off bills from the wedding?

An idea was born. It is only fair that the young couple agree to some sort of warranty on their marriage as a condition of securing the funding for the wedding. If they give up on the marriage before some reasonable date (that is, the end of the warranty period), they should pay back a portion of the expenses others incurred. Think about it, you wouldn't plunk down money for a washing machine without some sort of warranty that it was going to last for a few years. And if it stopped working after two or three loads, you'd expect to be able to get your money back. Of course, like tire tread, if it lasted pretty well but didn't quite live up to the warranty, you could live with a smaller refund. No one's trying to be unreasonable.

This next part is for accountants. Guys, the cost of the wedding could be amortized over, say, ten years, and the couples that don't make it will pay back the unamortized portion plus some reasonable rate of interest. Would LIBOR be acceptable?

It makes perfect sense. It should make couples think twice about giving up. Since it will be more expensive to divorce, it might even make people think more seriously about getting married. Wouldn't you pick your movies more carefully if you knew you couldn't easily leave in the middle?

It's all good except for one thing. The lovebirds who had decided they now could no longer coo on the same perch would never pay it back. Most likely they will be broke, but even if they weren't they would be in foul moods, and the expected response would be "It was his/her fault so get it from him/her." It is this shortcoming, however, that turns what was a smallish good idea into an economic tidal wave that would restore prosperity to the nation.

First of all, if there is a risk of non-payment, which there clearly is, the risk could easily be covered by a new form of insurance policy. Couples could obtain policies covering the repayment of their ceremony costs if the marriage went bust too quickly. In fact, similar to the procedure when one tries to obtain renewal of a license to drive, a routine question when one applied for a marriage license would be "All right, let me see photo identification and proof of insurance."

Insurance companies are like accountants without the sense of humor. To help them scientifically calculate the expected risks associated with the new policies, the industry would hire psychologists, marriage specialists, and members of other professions who probed the inner soul to help them grade the prospective couple's ability to stay married. One can imagine tearful scenes when the prospective bride and groom revealed that they had received very marginal grades. "Mommy, it's so unfair! They gave us a 4! [presumably a bad grade] Priscilla got a 5, and she told me that she was sleeping with the best man!" Weddings would be called off or delayed when grades were low.

Of course, given the importance of the scores, those gotta-get-good-grades types who were worried could sign up for marriage prep services where instructors would tutor applicants on how to do well on the exam. The insurance companies would also need investigators to prevent fraud. The criminal code would have to include something about marriage with the intent to divorce, to prevent those who would marry solely to try to collect the insurance policies. (It's ironic but it seems that many already do this, not realizing that there are not yet any policies on which to collect.)

What's the incentive for young married couples to stay together if they have insurance? By this time I expect you are answering the questions yourself. First there is the deductible—no deductible policies would just be too damn expensive. Second, try getting a policy in the future if one has been in too many previous mishaps. New Jersey has a thing called the state high cost pool for drivers too risky for the prudent insurance industry. It's very expensive. And, oh, the shame.

All of this makes sense and would have a dazzling effect on the economy. Marriages would last a bit longer, and some bad matches would never happen. The benefits of this for individual happiness would pale, however, in comparison to the benefits brought about by the bonanza of new jobs. These would be good, high paying professional jobs. Best of all, these jobs would be difficult to export. Who would want to calibrate risks of divorce using a marriage professional in China? I'm sure they are very smart over there, but the cultural divides would make it difficult for them to see what makes a young couple in Bellingham, Washington, a high-risk proposition. What could an insurance company do with a report that read: "Both man and woman seemed a bit silly and frivolous, but divorce is unlikely because she will be needed to pull the plow?"

Layer after layer of high paying jobs would be added to the economy. Apart from building another interstate highway system, or laying waste to the Alaskan wilderness, there really is nothing else that could generate as positive an economic punch as this. The political parties will wrangle for years before the politics are right to build more highways or to open Alaska to strip mining, so this idea really offers a unique opportunity for the political parties to agree and demonstrate that they can move the country forward.

So raise a glass and toast the happy couple, knowing that if you're lucky, and they are as incompatible as you think, you'll get your money back. You win either way: Either they are happy enough to stay together, or you get a windfall that you can use to fund a second honeymoon for yourself! Of course, if it isn't too selfish, let them enjoy themselves for a year or two and then develop irreconcilable differences. You really could use that second honeymoon.

At some point, my own marriage started to run into problems. Mary and I began to grow apart. I can't think of a particular triggering event. It just seemed to happen. Perhaps it was the health problems that each of us faced that began to preoccupy our attention. Whatever it was, I was the one to blink first. At a time when I did not know how long I had to find whatever it was that seemed to be missing, I moved out. To the surprise of many, we have tried to remain friends.

You may wonder why, given our separation, the interlude below about my wife and her battles with her health problems appears here rather than elsewhere. It belongs here because I wrote it as a love letter to her at a time when she thought I did not understand what she was going through. She felt alone. I was in California and wrote it through the night rather than sleeping, calling her first thing in her morning to tell her about it. My first title was "I'm in Love with a Crazy Lady," which offended her. Much has happened between us since then. The story changed as well. It was written to express love; it hopefully now will be accepted as a gift of great affection, and as a wake up call to others with bipolar mates who may have made the same mistakes I did.

Thirteenth Interlude:
The Bipolar Blues

Imagine if we blamed cancer victims for the fact that they were ill. Before claiming we never would, we must acknowledge that we once did. Though we now think of the Middle Ages as an unfortunate low point in our history, we can't deny their occurrence. And we sometimes act as if they never ended.

The Middle Ages were fertile soil for the growth of strange ideas. Times were tough, life was short, and there was little entertainment. Disease wiped out large chunks of humanity despite the fact that people crowded together in tightly packed churches to pray for deliverance. If God was good, all-powerful and loved them, why did such awful things keep happening?

The church had an answer. It also had an army. If you didn't have a bigger army, you accepted its answer. Bad things happened, the church said, because God gave man free will to choose between good and evil, and some men chose to follow evil. Disease was not sent by God, but caused by people embracing evil spirits. In other words, people "chose" to have the ailments that afflicted them. A good beating was thought a good cure because it could chase away the spirit causing the disease. Those people who lacked enough wit to pretend to be cured by the beating often were burned at the stake for harboring especially stubborn spirits.

We have made substantial progress in most areas since the Middle Ages. Our treatment of mental illness, however, sometimes makes one forget which century we are living in.

My wife has bipolar disorder. This disease, sometimes called "manic depression," causes its victims to cycle between periods of manic energy and debilitating depression.

Many of us unknowingly marvel at those with this ailment, witnessing only their "manic" sides. It doesn't seem to be a disease at all. What you observe is a wonderful, tireless and ingenious person. Many of the people we consider "great" (though not always "good") are thought to have been bipolar, including Napoleon, Alexander the Great, Alexander Hamilton, Abraham Lincoln and Winston Churchill. So too are a large number of leaders in business, the science and the arts.

But there is another side, rarely witnessed. The energy dissipates, the enthusiasm wanes, and a wave of depression so complete settles in that the individual who had been turning the world upside down now cannot get out of bed. Arms and legs still work, but the victim will lie staring into space without moving.

The cause of the offending behavior is molecular; it is caused by not having the right chemical stew in their brains. It is treatable, not by giving victims a good talking to, but by restoring the brain's correct chemistry. This understanding of the disease is recent. Most people, including many doctors, still respond to the disease as if the victim just needed to cheer up and get on with life.

I, with my Parkinson's disease, and my wife with her bipolar disorder, are a self-contained test bed to observe the different treatment accorded those whose ailments cause physical, or mental, symptoms.

I have received empathy and compassion. My wife has been treated less generously. People seemed to keep their distance from her. Many believed that she was at least partly responsible for her illness. I know this because I was often given credit by well-intentioned but ill-informed friends for putting up with her. I confess that at one time I joined them in thinking that she could just pick herself up and get on with it if she wanted.

Those with bipolar disorder do not choose to enter their periods of deep depression; the darkness wells up and overwhelms them. Yet, we treat them as if it were their fault, or as if they aren't really sick. Because my wife's chemistry affects her brain rather than her limbs, insurance companies seem to doubt that there is really a problem, and they reimburse treatment less completely than if, say, she were suffering from something "real" like tennis elbow.

Finding the right medicines to treat an individual's bipolar disorder is a matter of trial and error. Each new effort can be accompanied by side effects such as vomiting, sleeplessness, intestinal distress, weight gain or worse. It takes months to get it right, and because the body's needs change, getting it right is a never-ending process. Right today, wrong tomorrow. The fun never stops.

Doing this with one doctor is fun; doing it with more than one makes it exciting as well. Few doctors seem ready to adjust their thinking based on the experience or input of others. The patient gets to bounce from one treatment to another and back again, without the chance to discover if any of them work.

The result can be totally devoid of humor. A doctor practicing at a local hospital threatened my wife with involuntary commitment because she refused to take a drug he had prescribed. She had previously tried the drug while under the care of her own doctor, a psychiatrist with substantial experience in the area. It had caused severe muscular tremors, and he had taken her off the drug, concerned that continued use in her case could result in irreversible damage. The hospital doctor knew this. Yet he declined either to consult with her doctor or to change his proposed treatment.

The New Jersey legislature has considered a proposal that would provide doctors working with the mentally ill the right to request that a judge incarcerate patients who refused to take the medicines the doctors recommended! In light of my wife's experience, I can only view this with horror.

Many people don't do what their doctors recommend. What about smokers who keep smoking, heart patients who continue to overindulge in huge fatty steaks, diabetics who cannot give up candy, the elderly who drive when they can barely see their hands, and so on? Many of these groups are more dangerous or impose greater burdens on society than the mentally ill. Yet we think a person suffering depression should be locked up for ignoring his doctor, while an extremely overweight individual with a heart hanging on for dear life can "supersize" his meal at McDonald's with impunity.

Doctors who take the time to explain their proposed treatments to patients and their families rarely encounter patients unwilling to listen or take their medicine. Those doctors who don't communicate well with their patients may face greater problems. The right solution is to implant personalities into the doctors, not put their patients in jail.

Our treatment of those with mental illness no doubt contributes to the fact that between a quarter and a half of those diagnosed with bipolar disorder attempt suicide. About fifteen percent are "successful." These numbers remove any doubts that we are doing a good job for those who suffer this disease. We're not.

My wife's older brother is in those statistics. Raised by parents who were ashamed of his illness, and who assumed that he could "just get over it," he was never given proper medical treatment. (Our own attempts to intervene were too little, too late.) Instead, he lived in his parents' home, untreated, until age thirty-four when he killed himself. Had he suffered a physical ailment and been left untreated in his room, great attention would have been paid to this tragedy. But he died of mental illness, and the proper treatment is so little understood by most that neither the parents nor the community seemed to notice its absence.

There are increasing numbers of physicians treating bipolar disorder who know what they are doing. It is worth the effort to find them. My wife found several excellent doctors. She is back among the living because of them. It would not have been possible for those lacking the resources we have, however, to do what we did. Much of the treatment she obtained was not covered by insurance because many insurance carriers limit physician compensation for mental illness below that available for physical problems.

Those with bipolar disorder should not be disheartened. Nor should they settle for bad treatment. Find a doctor who knows what he's doing and put pressure on the insurance companies to pay him. It's your life, and it's worth fighting for.

If one you love has bipolar disorder, you need to understand what he or she is going through. If you don't, who will? *An Unquiet Mind*, a wonderful book by Kaye Redfield Jamison, is a good place to start. It is where I began, and I suspect I am not alone in owing her a debt of gratitude.

I hope that this has helped you begin to understand bipolar disorder, but that was not really my main purpose. I wrote this as a confirmation to my wife; a final exam to show her that I get it! I understand and accept your illness, including both the good and the bad that go with it. We will get through this!

By the way, there is something else we need to do. Our basement is a disaster. Any chance you feel a mania coming on so we can get it cleaned up? I would help, but unfortunately my symptoms are acting up and I'd better just relax and watch a ball game. If you finish early, let me know. I'm sure I'll feel better by the time you're done.

The rest of you with normal brains stay away from her—she's mine. Find your own "crazy lady" or clean your house yourself.

This is dedicated to the memory of Thomas Peter Gilroy, III, born February 25, 1959, died October 19, 1993.

☆ ☆ ☆

Too few of my stories begin as this one does, "I was in a bar in St. Thomas..." I remember this bar, at the Ritz Carlton, with great affection. On one visit, I was sitting and talking to a young bartender with whom I had become friendly when a young couple, very much in love, joined us at the bar.

The feelings of love that they had for each other were so visible that it broke through my layers of cynicism about relationships and made me realize how perfect life could be if one could capture and preserve the feelings that they had for each other. Yes they were newlyweds, but why must such feelings vanish with time? They wanted me to write about them, and I did. I hope what I wrote makes you feel that the search for what they had is worth the effort.

Fourteenth Interlude:

Love

I was in a bar in St. Thomas, talking to the bartender and listening to Louis Armstrong sing "What a Wonderful World," when a young couple sat down a few seats away. My bartender friend slid down to make them drinks, and I had the opportunity to observe them, which

I did without any effort to be discrete. Romantic music was in my ears, wine was in my blood, and the woman would have attracted the attention of a dead man. Her skin was tanned, and her blouse was low cut. (Ladies, take note. That combination is over-powering to those of us whose nature it is to adore you.) I looked again. Her blouse was no match for its occupants, which looked like they were going to escape at any moment.

The couple looked at each other rather than seeking out new faces. Their hands could not go for very long without finding an excuse to touch. It was enjoyable to see and reminded me of what it was like to be head over heels in love. The secret of their success: They had been married only two weeks. It struck me that their coming to the bar and engaging in conversation was a little like going into the kitchen for a snack during halftime. They were taking a break from each other and gathering their strength. I was the halftime entertainment. Well, one shouldn't disappoint.

We traded polite questions of each other. He was an auto mechanic, she a kindergarten teacher. Both were from Minnesota. I said that I was a writer. They asked me to write about them, with all the trusting innocence that people from places like Minnesota seem to have. I asked what would make them noteworthy or unique. Their answer, delivered with the confidence of those too young to have experienced many failures, was that they intended to stay in love. They were confident, the woman explained, because they had waited to make love until marriage, and on marriage until they had found their soul mates. I quickly glanced at the man as she said this. Unlike her other remarks, which he had generally echoed with words or gestures of agreement, he greeted this statement with a concentrated draw on his beer, eyes down.

The linkage between postponing sex and extending love is a core belief held by many. I've never understood the logic. Abstinence causes men to act very confused, or to think we see God, and it's very difficult to tell while we're in that state what we will be like when sexual activity ceases to be a preoccupation. For better or worse, we act differently once this aspect of the relationship ensues. It is less risky to decide whether you like us *after* we've changed into what we're really like than before.

Man's constant readiness to fulfill his sexual mission does not mean that he doesn't also want love. I found myself hoping that these two really would maintain a love for each other. Most couples don't manage it. When I thought of my friends and acquaintances, I could think of only a very small minority who had not divorced. An even smaller number of those still married were still in love.

Perhaps we don't remember how wonderful love is. Seeing these two drown in each other's eyes brought back how intense the feelings could be. Ah, to be in love. It was a wonderful feeling that was much too scarce.

Allow me to pry into all of our childhoods to try to remind you of what "love" can be. Do you remember having what as adults we disparagingly refer to as a "crush?" While our adult perception is that this was something less than mature love, it in fact remains for most people an illustration of the power and intensity of "love" in its most uncomplicated form. Having a crush was the surest way of replacing your stomach with an empty void that ached until you discovered whether your love was welcome, and returned. Not only did you lose a stomach, but also your brain could think of nothing else except that your happiness depended on the answer.

The moment of truth would arrive with overwhelming impact. Most of my experiences ended with intense but temporary feelings of disappointment and despair. But there were also times when childish infatuation was rewarded with the revelation that the object of my desire was just as nervously hoping that I returned her feelings towards her! She likes me! We like each other! The feeling following the discovery of love was intense. Walking was easy because your feet didn't touch the ground. It was pure joy. Yes, it passed. Yes, it was less robust than the adult version that added sexual complications, mortgages, careers and children into the mix. It was wonderful.

When was the last time you experienced love so intense that you couldn't eat? I congratulate those of you who can remember. Too few will answer: "Today!" Why?

I remain utterly fascinated with evolution as a starting point to understand the human condition. Everything we are, everything we do, is derived from some chance mutation that helped those affected survive and reproduce. If a trait were merely noble or wonderful but didn't create an edge in the battle for survival, there would be no reason it would be sustained. Underlying every soft sentiment, every act of selflessness, is a reason as brutal in competitive effect as the development of the opposable thumb. Love might not have enabled us to grasp weapons more effectively as did the thumb. But the fact that the emotion is still with us means that those who were capable of it were more capable of surviving and outlasting those who weren't.

The fact that love can make us feel ecstatic is very revealing. The euphoria it produces is evidence of its importance to our survival. Things that were very important to the survival of the species (such as love and sex) are rewarded with intense pleasure; things that are very bad for the survival of the species (such as being eaten by a crocodile) are punished with severe pain. Not trusting that we would do what was best for ourselves without incentives, evolution produced survivors with built in carrot-and-stick guidance systems to help them navigate the dangers of uncivilized life. Euphoria is the ultimate reward our bodies can pay our minds, reserved for actions so important to our survival that nature tries to make sure that we don't neglect them.

It is easy to see how love was necessary to the survival of creatures having the reproductive characteristics of humans. Let us suppose that men cared nothing for the women with whom they were making babies. (Now ladies, if you still have this complaint, you chose poorly. There are men who do care.) In uncivilized times, when surviving the day really meant surviving the day, being pregnant was more of an issue than simply being uncomfortable. Pregnancy made the woman increasingly vulnerable. It is tough to run from danger when you are eight months pregnant.

Before the advent of love, the appearance of a predator would have caused an "every man for himself" flight for safety. The attrition rate of pregnant women and the small children who did manage to be born would have been very high. Pregnancy would slow the women down and make them less able to defend themselves when caught. Children are natural born appetizers. Unlike some species, in which a two- or three-year-old can bring down a wildebeest, human children are pretty useless in a fight for years after birth. Without an incentive for others to protect them, the women and children would keep getting picked off. The group's chances for survival would be nothing to write on cave walls about.

When that wonderful mutation occurred that suffused the men with a desire to protect women and children, the beginnings of what we call love was born. Those men who felt good when they protected their mates and offspring triumphed, because their mates and offspring were far more likely to have descendants who would perpetuate that genetic trait. Love came to town and was here to stay.

The emotion needed to be intense to be effective. Feeling "kind of good" about protecting women and children wouldn't really cut it. It could not have been an easy decision to stop and face the pursuing beast, risking a horrible death. The man facing the charging lion needed to feel more than modestly interested in protecting his "family," because another part of his brain was sending messages based on the instinct for survival. As the lion got closer and closer, the man's brain was being bombarded on the one hand with this new "love" thing and on the other with an old familiar voice of survival, saying something like: "What are you, nuts? That's a lion coming at you, asshole! Run for it! So what if it eats your children? You can always make more!"

Those whose genetic make-up produced only mild stirrings of love would almost certainly have succumbed to such talk. These men would have run for their lives, hoping that the lion would be distracted by munching on the pregnant woman and whatever children were around as long as possible, giving him enough time to escape.

Eventually heroes would be born who felt such bonds of love towards their mates and their progeny that they would protect them even at great personal risk. Those who were brave and noble but not very clever at fighting off predators were soon killed off. Contrary to popular song, love was not all that was needed. Love and the ability to kill or chase away lions were needed. Those who had all these traits were our ancestors.

Woman's love of man followed the same trail. The woman who developed the capability to love would increase her mate's and her own chances for survival. Though not as strong as the man, she was able to watch his back, perhaps taking turns standing guard, perhaps nursing him back to health after some mishap, or perhaps using greater intelligence than he possessed to figure a way out of some jam. Such activity would sometimes put her at risk as well, requiring a good deal of courage to "stand by her man."

The love that was carved into our genetic code has its limitations, however. We may aspire to maintain love "till death do us part," but that is not the love evolution handed off to us. In the battle for survival, the woman was not worth defending once she could have no more children and had finished caring for those that she had had. After that point, no matter how wonderful a person she was, she became expendable. Men whose genetic make-up made them love their mates till that point, and then transfer their affections to younger females, were likely to sire more children than the mate we would call faithful. There is certainly no reason why our social conventions need to be patterned after the behavior of men at the time when we lived in caves. But permanency, while a desired attribute of love, is not an inherent part of our genetic programming.

While the above reasoning is theoretical, it also seems logical. Besides, it's not as if we are totally lacking a window that enables us to get an empirical glimpse of what we were like millions and millions of years ago. There are places in this world, and even in this country, where man's progress has been so stunted that our distant past has been preserved as a living laboratory, illustrating what people were like in prehistoric times. I won't identify any locations at this time for fear of causing offense. Suffice it to say that the areas in the United States where such backward circumstances remain voted Republican in the last presidential election.

Let us return to the bar. Our young couple is intensely in love and determined to be different from all those who start out in love but end bitter or, worse, numb and disinterested.

How can couples maintain the wonderful feelings of love with which they set out on their life adventure? We cannot simply rely on nature to take its course, because our evolutionary programming allows love to fade with time. Yet these young love birds were persuaded by the heat of their passion that their love would outlast their lust and end only with their death.

I wanted it to happen. I wanted to tell them that the most important thing is, as the song says, to "shower the people you love with love" and to let them know how you feel by a thousand little things. I realized that I would sound like a sentimental drunk so I hemmed and hawed.

They asked for their check and began to make preparations to leave. As they started to stand up, I stood up to say goodbye, but instead found myself asking if I could say something before they left. They paused and I began: "I really hope you do stay in love your entire lives. Some people do, although it's rare. I will write about you, but I want you to promise me one thing: If you start feeling that your love is slipping, I want you to go to the zoo, go to the lions' cage and watch the lions." Looking at the woman, I added, "Don't ask me how I know, but he loves you so much he would fight that animal if necessary to protect you. Remember that."

I then turned to the man and said, "And she loves you enough that she would weep at your funeral and miss you terribly, because you don't appear capable of surviving an encounter with the average lion. If by some miracle you do survive, she will try to stitch what's left of you together. Remember that."

I know these words were a little short of the profundity you expected. They certainly didn't have the desired effect on the couple, who looked puzzled, said a quick goodbye, and excused themselves. Hey, I had drunk quite a bit, and it was the best I could do with so little time to think. Still, I had no doubt that they would remember the story about the zoo. And I wrote this story as promised in the hope they would read it and find here the words I wished I had said.

The conversation also made me decide to go back to my room, although it was almost a certainty that my own wife would be asleep. At the very least, I wanted to make sure that she was safe. The problem with modern love, I decided, was that you seldom encountered wild animals at the Ritz, and it was all too easy to forget what we would do for each other if we were put to the test. I would at least make certain she had sun block for tomorrow.

My thanks to the couple from Minnesota who reminded me of what it was like to be head over heels in love.

☆ ☆ ☆

My son, a product of my first marriage, is grown. He is now a friend, fast on his way to becoming the father figure in our relationship. He is very mature; I have chosen to reject maturity. He is responsible; I remember when I was. Been there; done that.

My daughter appears willing to permit me to continue being her parent a bit longer, although I get the raised eyebrows and the "Daa-a-ad" drawl when I become too silly. Still, she lights up my life as no one else can by greeting me with hugs and adoration when I come through the door, and sincere wails of "don't go" when I leave. A smile from her makes me feel ten feet tall. She smiles a lot, and it is getting difficult to find clothes that fit.

I moved out of our home because I reached a point in my life where I wanted to be whatever I needed to be to have the fun I delayed too many times in the past. The fear of not living long enough to enjoy the store of nuts I kept saving for a rainy day, or worse, being an invalid unable to gather rosebuds or do much of anything else, motivated me to explore new territory where I could eat nuts, gather rosebuds and try to find happiness. I regret the pain I caused my wife and daughter, and I hope someday they will forgive me, even if my daughter may not understand these words now.

Despite no longer living in the same house, I try to see my daughter as much as possible. I can't imagine life without her, and I will never understand those parents who are cruel to their children. That doesn't mean one doesn't have difficult times, or that I enjoy every minute we are together. There are times where enjoyment is hard to find.

School science fairs are among those times, at least for me. I told my daughter's teacher, an absolutely wonderful woman named Ms. Sharma, that I had written about the science fair held during my daughter's second grade year. We discussed how much it had improved for her third grade. I agreed. Ms. Sharma then asked what nice things I was going to say, to give my description of the previous year "balance." This was said with the usual twinkle in her eye. She followed with a promise to buy a copy of this book, and I promised her, like so many others, the very first copy printed. Ms. Sharma, the balance is this: You are the best teacher my daughter has had or I suspect ever will have. You not only love to teach, but you love my daughter as much as I think you would if she were yours. If only every parent could feel that way about their children's teachers. Thank you!

Now you must take the bad with the good…

FIFTEENTH INTERLUDE:
WHY I HATE SCIENCE FAIRS

One night a year I spend a miserable evening with my daughter. I love my daughter and almost always have a wonderful time with her. She's seven, an age where little girls still love and admire their fathers. It's a perfect age with neither diapers nor boyfriends. How can any time with her be less than pure joy? It is the night of the science fair, the night the children present the results of the projects they have performed in order to get "hands on" scientific experience. It's not a bad idea, or wouldn't be if you kidnapped the parents and held them until it was over.

I attended the science fair for my daughter's second grade class this week. The rows of exhibits contained one sophisticated display after another, dealing with such typical second grade interests as logic gates, thermodynamics and organic chemistry. I at first thought that these must be very talented second graders. But as I watched for a few more minutes, the truth began to emerge. The kids were running around, chasing each other, giggling and going to the few tables that had "fun" things to do. One exhibit, which made their hair stand on end with electricity, was particularly popular. For the most part, though, the children were oblivious to the projects, for the simple reason that the projects were too advanced to arouse the interest of a seven-year-old.

When did the children become irrelevant at science fairs? Tell the truth: How many of you have done the science projects your kids were supposed to do? I plead guilty of this crime in the past, but I am now reformed, and like most who recover from some affliction, I am evangelical about helping others avoid making the same mistake. Most of us have done our children's projects for them at some point. It's really not hard to tell.

The projects done by kids are generally simple experiments, explained on poster boards in words that either slope up or slope down. That doesn't mean the projects aren't good; it means they were made by children. At their best, the genuine child-produced projects exhibit childish fascination with scientific topics that are part of their world—things that they can see or touch or smell.

The parents' projects, in contrast, are about underlying forces or properties of nature of which the children are unaware. The words are neatly scribed in straight lines or appear in separate computer-generated handouts. The explanations I read didn't help me. I am a retired lawyer, which puts my scientific understanding at about a sixth grade level. Okay, a fifth grade level. I figured I had three grade levels on these kids so I would be able to hold my own. I didn't understand most of the projects, and I suspect that many of the seven-year-olds didn't either. What is the fun in that?

Parents also get carried away at their children's athletic events, yelling at coaches and referees, and exhorting their children to knock the seven- or eight-year-olds on the opposing team "on their butts." At least with athletics, though, the parents are not permitted to take the field and play for their children. For whatever reason, however, the parents are allowed to "take the field" at science fairs, often becoming the actual presenter of their, ahem, child's work.

Parents with engineering and science backgrounds rarely have opportunities to put their substantial talents on public display. They aren't very good in athletics because they ruined their vision studying late at night. Nor are they the center of attention at parties or used to being in the spotlight. The science fair is one of the few opportunities where they are in their natural element. Their desire to show off a bit at science fairs is understandable, but unacceptable. This is their children's opportunity, and the parents should not deprive them of it.

We need to get the parents "off the field." Science is as important as sports, and we ought to give our kids a chance to roll around in it, and enjoy it. How do we gracefully move the parents to the side without offense? We don't want them to lose interest, because they are brainy people who can help the children learn. They just need a little coaching as to how.

First, teachers should assign the projects. Parents, if given free reign, will pick something that they are familiar with, perhaps related to their occupation. With a little creativity with topic selection, we can remove whatever interest they may have had in taking over either the preparation or presentation of the report.

Projects involving human bodily functions will fascinate the children while making the parents squirm. Most adults are very uncomfortable talking publicly about such things. That makes topics like the human digestive system and excretory functions perfect areas to explore, a veritable gold mine of ideas that will interest the children while keeping the parents at bay.

For example, one could explore the effects of different foods on the digestive system, measured by the gas that each causes the body to produce. Students could select three or four different foods with lots of fiber. Baked beans would certainly be a good candidate. Guests at the fair would be assigned to groups and would eat one of the foods when they first arrived at the fair. Then about a half an hour later they could be observed to determine whether some foods caused more flatulence than others. The students could graph the response times and severity levels to compare how the body coped with one food group versus another. There is a great deal of science that could be learned in the process, and you'd have to beat the kids with a stick to stop them from learning it. The parents would do just about anything to avoid being associated with the project, or the resulting papers: "The Process of Gas Propagation in a Closed Environment" and "Exploring the Food Chain: the Effects of Fiber on the Digestive Process." Perfect.

What about a study of phlegm? The good thing about this one is that no matter when the fair is held, there is always at least one child producing this substance in commercial quantities. The kids could learn why the body produces phlegm and measure the effects on its production of different foods, such as dairy products. Of course it's gross to most of us; but that just makes it more fascinating to children. Who wants to participate in "The Effect of Dairy Products on the Production of Phlegm in Seven-Year-Olds?"

We are wasting a golden opportunity to make our children fascinated with science. We should be helping them use scientific methods to study their world, not making their first experiences with science frustrating by talking about things they don't care about and don't understand! There isn't a second grader in the world who wouldn't rather talk about farting than logic gates. By using topics that are meaningful to them to teach them science, we can channel their fascination into scientific curiosity. If you want them to love science, start with farts and snot; not thermodynamics.

We have a choice: Interest them in science, and we can lay the groundwork for a scientific renaissance; continue as we are, and while we continue to lag in science, we should have large numbers of children interested in becoming lawyers and investment bankers. They can always buy Japanese and German cars if our engineering doesn't improve!

PART IX:

Life requires a change of scenery every once in a while. There is something about the demands of work and family that make it essential to escape to some place that gives you the courage to keep trying to do the impossible and satisfy all the demands put on you in your everyday-life at home.

The recuperative purpose of vacations makes it all the more important that vacations be successful. If a vacation disappoints and adds rather than reduces stress, then it becomes doubly depressing. Fortunately, those who help us with our vacations know this. Airlines make certain we are whisked to our destinations on time, in comfort, and have our luggage waiting for us without fail when we arrive. It was confirmation of their great concern for our safety and enjoyment that led to this next interlude, written after I had the pleasure of flying across country in a middle seat, with a bag of peanuts and a cup of bad coffee for nourishment.

SIXTEENTH INTERLUDE:
ARE PEOPLE GETTING SMALLER OR ARE THE AIRLINES MISINFORMED?

Watching professional sports can educate as well as entertain. Anyone who has watched basketball or football knows the answer to the question posed by the title. People are not getting smaller; on average, we're getting bigger. Compare the sizes of players in the National Basketball Association who played thirty years ago to those playing today. The guards of today are nearly the size of the earlier centers. There was a time when a seven-foot player was a wonder of nature; now every team has one or two.

Football too shows an increase in size. Three hundred pound players were once considered aberrations; now if a lineman doesn't weigh at least that much, he is considered undersized. Quarterbacks are much bigger too, so they can see over the linemen. Many are well over six feet tall. Even today's cheerleaders are bigger than Fran Tarkenton, a diminutive quarterback who played successfully for the Minnesota Vikings and other teams years ago.

The increased size of athletes is not a secret. Nor is it unique. People are larger than the men and women of earlier times. It's not because we drink milk; it's because the mating choices appear to favor those who are tall rather than short. That's not a problem unless you happen to be short. The rest of us can adjust quite nicely to longer limbs. Clothing manufacturers can be informed. We don't have to walk around with sleeves that are too short. We buy shirts with longer sleeves. Car manufacturers notice; they build cars with more headroom. In fact, there is only one institution that seems to be misinformed about, or ignores, the size of their customers: the airlines.

Given the amount of interaction they have with the public, how do the airlines arrive at the conclusion that people are shrinking? It's pretty tough. They even fly the athletes around, for crying out loud! Don't they notice that they are bigger than they used to be? They seem to think the opposite.

Each new interior design of the airplanes they introduce provides less space per passenger than its predecessor. Seats are significantly less wide than they once were, so that a passenger carrying extra pounds no longer fits within his own space. The ceiling height of newer planes, particularly those designed in Brazil, is comfortable if you are no larger than Tattoo (of *Fantasy Island* fame), but otherwise makes you stoop every time you try to stand up.

No one complains! Why? Because if you do, your name is taken and you are likely to find on your next flight that you have been assigned to a middle seat, a fate nice people don't wish on their worst enemy. You think the airlines don't play games with seat assignments? Then tell me why, as surely as night follows the day, those people with weak bladders are given window seats. No, these folks at the airlines know what they are doing.

If you're thin, with good posture and short legs, you can just fit into a middle seat. A variation of any of these attributes and you're in trouble. Even if you fit, though, you quickly realize that there is no room to move during the flight. Of course you have to stuff your carry-on under the seat in front of you, because the luggage bins, which are designed to hold the possessions of about half the number of passengers that the plane carries, are full. There is now no room for your feet, so your knees are pushed back towards your ears.

Just as you calm yourself using the deep breathing technique you learned in yoga, you see the two wide-bodies being escorted to the seats on either side of you.

I don't mean to pick on overweight people. I feel sorry for the embarrassment this situation must cause them. Their excess poundage is made all too obvious because it will not fit into their space, which means it must spill into yours. On flights where it gets a little warm, you are pinned motionless, and the parts of your side in contact with your neighbors become wet with perspiration. They're not bad people and I suspect this causes them mental stress.

They suffer the same as the person in the window seat who is bladder challenged and has just asked you to move, even though you can't, so he can go to the bathroom for the sixth time since you left Newark an hour ago. You look hopefully at the passenger with the aisle seat, but he's ticked at the constant interruptions, so he's pretending to be asleep. This forces Mr. Bladder-About-to-Burst to slide out to the aisle, crushing your knees and keeping his posterior in your face for a dangerously long period of time. Sometimes you're lucky, sometimes you're not.

At least the airlines are trying to help. Most of them have stopped giving food during flights to help their passengers lose weight. But their efforts are too little too late. Many of their passengers are already too large, and making them go hungry doesn't fix the problem in a useful time frame.

What would you do if a manufacturer of clothes ignored reality the way airlines do and made their clothes smaller each year, so that your arms would only be covered two-thirds by the sleeves and the waist fasteners wouldn't quite fasten? You'd buy your clothes elsewhere. So why don't you do the same with air travel? Aha! It's equally obvious: Nine times out of ten you have no choice between what I just described and something better.

If those two points are true, and they are, the current deregulatory framework isn't working as hoped. *Shirt makers make clothes that fit because you have choice; airlines make seats that don't fit because you don't.* Competition has failed to flourish, allowing airlines to abuse their customers with impunity. And it appears that some of them quite enjoy it. Forgive me, Mr. Kahn, but this isn't what you had in mind, is it? Shouldn't we take another look?

For the last several years, as my Parkinson's has advanced, I have been getting massages to help keep my muscles loose. Why would I ever give my masseuse, a very nice young lady, reason to attack my knotted muscles with more vigor than she already does? Yet, when she shared that she and her husband were planning a vacation and that she was concerned about what might happen to her little dog in the kennel while they were gone, I couldn't help myself. I started immediately composing this story out loud to tease her, causing her to do an excellent job of assuring that none of those muscle knots survived.

She also changed her plans and decided not to put her dog in the kennel. Instead she found someone who loves pets as much as she does to watch her dog in her home. It seems unfair that I should benefit from my bad behavior, but I now use the same person to watch my dog Coop, even though, as I explain, Coop really could fend for herself.

The reason I have given up on kennels is quite different. Coop is the only dog I've had that gets car sick. She gets *very* car sick. Immediately upon entering the car, she starts drooling excessively. I'm talking about gallons of the stuff. At the twenty-minute mark, if you have not reached your destination, she looks at you with her big brown eyes and starts the dry heaves that are a certain precursor to her throwing up. Because the eyes and mouth face in the same direction, I have no choice but to try to push her sad face away from me.

My worst trip to the kennel occurred as a result of waiting until the last minute to make a reservation for Coop. Every kennel within a twenty minute radius, what I call drool-only range, was full. I boarded her at one about thirty-five minutes away, clearly post-drool, and likely multiple-vomit territory. She rewarded me by throwing up an even half dozen times on the way, looking at me with her big sad eyes each time.

What could I do? I cleaned up the car as best I could and gave it to my son as his college graduation present.

SEVENTEENTH INTERLUDE:

FUN IN THE SUN; TERROR IN THE KENNEL

I had a young friend, an attractive lady, who had two loves: her husband and her terrier of some sort or other. At home her heart was big enough to caress both with all the hugs and kisses they could want, and indeed neither one was or needed to be jealous of the other. Each received a different type of affection, and each liked what they received and wouldn't have traded places for the world. The puppy often wondered how the man could look so content without being scratched behind the ears. Humans are very strange and easily pleased, he thought. (I realize the skeptics among you have inched forward on their haunches, ready to pounce. "How does he know what a dog was thinking?" Listen, this story wouldn't have been written without a lot of after-the-fact interviews with those involved. I know what I know.)

The equilibrium did not apply outside the home. There, time spent with one meant time not spent with the other. Earlier that spring, with her nesting instincts unconsciously driving her actions, the woman began gathering flyers for one beach resort after another. These places, where little was worn and there was even less to do, had a demonstrated track record with the male of the species. Take away his friends, beer and football, and put him in an environment where he is surrounded by bare legs, nearly bare breasts and deceptively strong rum drinks, and it is not even a fair fight. He will do everything in his power to make love to his wife, without a thought about family planning. Previous concerns about being too young to start the years of changing diapers, working to pay for college, or chewing his nails when he sees his son's nose ring or daughter's skimpy clothes are no match for the devil's brew he is now confronting.

It's not that the man wouldn't have chosen to do the exact same thing if he had been allowed to think with his head, but he was not. It is a fact, or at least sounds like it should be, that when a woman's total wardrobe weighs three ounces or less, a man's brain is not permitted to participate in any decisions made with respect to her. At somewhere around five ounces of clothes, men regain their power of speech, but still can't say anything that makes any sense. Somewhere near a pound of clothing, men start slouching, scratching their bellies or butts, and shouting from whatever room they happen to be in, "Honey, I'm hungrier than hell. Can you hurry and get dinner on the table. I'm going bowling tonight, and you know how long it takes to digest your cooking."

Each brochure sounds and looks great. The resort owners, who know exactly what's going on, cater to the real decision makers. Little touches like fresh flowers in tasteful china vases help bait the trap. The men focus solely on whether the brochure mentions parasailing until they are there and it's too late.

To the woman, there is only one thing that isn't absolutely perfect, and that is the policy, in unobtrusive type on the second page, which says "no pets." Someday she will find a place that allows both pets and husbands. Together they offer a complete package; separately they reveal their distinct weaknesses. Men are good at translating affection into sexual energy, but are lousy at offering warmth and affection for extended periods. Pets offer unlimited love and affection. Their only desire is to be with you. Yet once they finish the mandatory slobber and drool, they are not really as good a source of romance as are men, on those nights when there is nothing good on television.

As the time for their vacation grows near, the need to find a place for the dog to stay for a week or so grows more urgent. The woman had collected brochures on these places too, but they all seemed lacking.

Finally, she selected the one that was most expensive. She thought, and of course the kennel owners knew her thinking, that the higher price must mean that the care was better. If not, it was hard to understand how the price charged to stay in the kennel—a cheaply constructed structure of unpainted concrete blocks, mesh fencing and stained concrete floors—could be nearly as much as their deluxe room.

It was not as if every animal could get in! The new kennel philosophy was that all dogs were put in a large pen together so that they could socialize. To that end, dogs had to come for pre-admittance interviews to show that they were not ruthless sociopaths. Of course the woman's dog passed with flying colors. It was shy and sweet, having lived all the life it could remember in an environment of love and pampering, where its needs were met before it realized it had them. I truly hate the use of foreshadowing in literature, but I feel compelled to mention that the pampering that made the dog feel so loved at home was ill preparation for life in the brutal world of the kennel.

The day of the vacation finally arrived, and, with tears and kisses, the woman left her little terrier at the kennel and drove to the airport with her husband. Left with the dog were several chew bones, a large bag of the most expensive dog food, and a toy or two. Just in case. The assistants in the front office of the kennel were dressed in matching uniforms and promised that the dog would have a vacation to remember!

The following accounts of the woman's time at the resort, and the dog's in the kennel, were pieced together from a variety of interviews with man and beast. In order to keep the narrative style, I have filled in some of the missing blanks, but always in a manner consistent with the way I felt like making them up.

The divergence of experiences didn't take long to develop. Upon arrival, the woman and her husband were greeted by a number of attractive and barely clothed employees of the resort. They were cheered, offered complimentary rum drinks, and then shown the resort's main attractions. They were finally shown to their room, a sunny affair with marble bathroom floors, a beautiful king size bed, and, of course, freshly cut flowers. They were tipsy by the time they were left alone. They began changing into their swimsuits when the man looked at his half clothed wife, threw his suit across the room and changed their immediate itinerary.

Let's leave this slice of heaven for a few minutes to check in on the young terrier, who, with a clean coat and not a worry in his head, set foot in the kennel for a week of playing with other dogs. He had a moment to wonder what games they might play before he saw a grey blur out of the corner of his eye, and felt himself being knocked painfully off his feet and into the fence. There must be some mistake. He waited for an apology. "Your food is mine," said a voice. He sensed another attack from behind before it happened and dodged just in time. Pretty lady, why did you do this to me?

A friendlier voice called to him. "That was a nice move, newbie. Come on over here. I can't promise you that you'll get your own food because the big dogs take all the expensive stuff, but stick with us and you'll get three squares a day and you'll live." The small dog walked over and found himself in the company of other small dogs. All of them were battle scarred, but morale was good. The small dog felt a little better and, switching to an inter-breed dialect, he began trying to make sense of things.

"I don't understand. I thought every dog was tested to see if they were friendly to other dogs."

"That's true," a small schnauzer answered, "But your people went away in off season." The terrier looked puzzled so the schnauzer explained,

"During off season, not as many people travel, so the kennel runs short of owners wanting to board their pets. To keep occupancy high, they grade on the curve." The terrier still looked a bit confused. "The curve?" he asked. The schnauzer replied, "It means that every dog passes, regardless of his record. So watch out, it's a dog eat dog world in here."

This was a tough message for an animal that was used to being woken up by a gentle voice saying "Is schnookems ready for breakfast?" The dog rubbed his eyes with his paws, half thinking that when he stopped and cleared his vision, all this ugliness would be gone. No luck. Then he looked for the well-dressed human attendants. They were talking on telephones or among themselves. He could also tell that, like most humans, these had not been "fixed" and they would therefore be playing their funny pre-mounting games. They would be of little use for years. For the life of him, he couldn't understand why the older humans didn't neuter some of the youngsters. You could tell by looking at them that some of them would never win a ribbon nor would they sire any winners. Why humans, who understood so well how to breed superior dogs, seemed content to produce such weak human specimens was a total mystery.

The immediate question was how to survive the week. He made friends with a few of the feistier small dogs, and they banded together swearing to defend each other to the death. The only place they could find in the kennel that looked like it offered defensible terrain was a corner away from the building where the fence pinched in a bit so that those seeking to attack this space would be squeezed together into a narrower funnel than the defenders. That offered some advantage, although being away from the building meant exposure without protection to the weather. Well, raindrops didn't bite. They moved out to their new space and watched for attacks around the clock.

Do you really want to hear any more about the humans? Let's see, after relaxing in their room for three or four hours, they went to dinner. Both enjoyed the six course tasting menu, with a different wine paired with each course They started with oysters, accompanied by the obligatory oyster jokes; moved to a tri-color salad made with a very fine, thinly sliced Parmesan; experimented with a pate which both decided to skip; wolfed down some scallops richly scented with garlic and olive oil, followed by a small but tasty tenderloin; and finally partook of a black and white chocolate mousse cake with a lattice of mint chocolate. It was all they could do to get enough exercise so that they didn't gain weight. They had a snorkeling adventure in the morning, and he signed up for parasailing the following day. And so it went.

That is as far as I will recount the details of the week. The dog's days were filled with fears, heroic battles and hunger. The people's days were filled with love, fine food and relaxation. It is a human's life, as dogs say.

All good things must come to an end, and the day came when the couple returned home. They had been expected the following morning, and the surprising timing caught the attendants spending a good deal of time and energy playing with each other while largely ignoring the pets. Disgusted, the woman pushed back the attendant and stepped into the kennel. And a good thing it was that she entered when she did. The little dogs were defending their fortress valiantly but were under ferocious assault by the larger and stronger dogs. The woman didn't hesitate. She picked up a stainless steel choke collar still attached to a leash, and using it like the reasonable imitation of a mace that it was, swung it and connected with loud thwacks against some of the larger dogs' heads. Like most bullies, the large dogs hadn't actually thought about getting hurt themselves. When it happened, they didn't like it, and they ran, whimpering, to the farthest corners of the kennel, to growl at this strange person hitting them.

The same experience can teach different lessons to different people, or dogs. The woman here was not a crusader, and having encountered a situation she did not like, she determined to avoid it in the future. They took no more vacations without the dog. Or their child. Yes, they have a little boy now. No, he did not result from this trip. After the trip, however, the woman fell into the habit of absent-mindedly scratching behind her husband's ears while they were watching television. That seemed to work as well as a tropical island. Actually, it seemed to work better. Try it; dogs have kept this secret to themselves for too long!

As for the terrier, he learned to appreciate that which he already had but had previously taken for granted. He is now a popular speaker at dog gatherings and has completely recovered from his experience. He is just a much quieter dog than he used to be.

There are several lessons one can draw from this story. Perhaps it has no lesson for you because the kennel you use is different. The little dog told me while I was taking notes on this story that word was there was a great kennel upstate somewhere, close to Canada. That may be the one you use. Or you can come to the same conclusion as the young woman here and decide to forego vacations that require boarding your dog.

As for me, I needed a solution that permitted me to go to the islands. I love it there. Besides that's where I write much of this stuff. I too have a dog and wouldn't want to worry that I would be subjecting her to bad treatment at the hands, that is to say, paws of the kennel ruffians.

Allow me to introduce Coop, my dog. Correction, my daughter's dog. She is a big dog. She is a strong dog. She is a smart dog. I suppose she has those traits one would expect from a mixed lab-shepherd-rottweiler who spent some time in a shelter as a puppy. While fun loving and slow to anger, she also has a growl that translates loosely in dog words as: "You talking to me?" You don't want to mess with Coop.

When I first heard what had happened to the terrier, I had a momentary panic. I took Coop for a walk, or more accurately she took me. As I massaged my aching muscles from the battles we had when she saw a squirrel or deer or other early rising human, I came to a calming conclusion: I'm not the one who has to worry.

You want to take vacations? Get a big dog.

PART X:

Politics And Death

If you've read this far, you don't offend easily. Like a drunk riding a mechanical bull in a bar, you have held on thus far without really understanding what you get for doing so. No rewards yet—you've not made it to the end. Let's see if we can't throw a few more off the bull before revealing the meaning of life in the epilogue!

What better way to serve that purpose than to talk in more detail about politics and death. Based on the close results of most elections, politics is a dangerous topic to pick—both liberal and conservative politicians generally attract close to half of the electorate, meaning that taking either side is likely to alienate about half of the potential readers out there. I can only hope that those who might be offended have already paid for this book, and that you are not still standing in the bookstore seeing whether you can finish it before that nosy sales person wonders what you have been doing for the last five hours. Moreover, I have decided to discuss a relatively safe topic to avoid stirring up those who might wish to do me harm—how to achieve peace in the Middle East.

Eighteenth Interlude:

Peace

People in the Middle East have lived in a world of unremitting conflict for thousands of years. That makes them serious. It's not that they never laugh; they do. But one must tread warily if one is going to discuss current events. Write something that offends people elsewhere and you get a nasty comment or two; here you get a bounty put on your head.

I woke up one day and felt that I had some role to play in the drama. Why not? I had the advantage of being almost totally ignorant of the issues. I also had an illness likely to reduce my life-expectancy, and was counting on the assumption that the regional terrorists would have certain minimum standards that would prevent them from wasting a martyr on someone moving along so quickly without their help. I also lacked plans for the coming weekend. The situation was tailor-made for me.

As luck would have it, the paper had a story about a hermit living in Central Park who claimed to be descended from Moses. I sought him out and asked him why God just didn't make the parties enter into a lasting peace. He loves both sides, and can do whatever He wants. The hermit looked at me, cocked his head as if listening to a voice I couldn't hear, and responded enigmatically, "Read Exodus."

I hadn't read the Bible for many years and did so now with very little hope of finding anything that spoke usefully to the current day. I was wrong. I discovered a God who was almost human—passionate and capable of anger when people failed to live up to His expectations. Oppose Him and He could become exasperated past the point of pulling His punches. When He became angry, He being God, all hell broke loose.

You think I exaggerate? Read Exodus! This God was a Supreme Being on a rampage! The story begins simply enough. The Jews were in trouble once again, this time as slaves in Egypt. God rolled His eyes thinking He couldn't turn his back without His chosen people getting in trouble. So He sent help—a man named Moses. The man looked surprisingly like Charlton Heston, the first hint that something was wrong. Whoever heard of a white man named Moses? Seth or Judah would have been believable. But a white man named Moses? You knew there was going to be trouble.

Moses told Pharaoh to let the Jews go. Pharaoh declined. Now, before you think that Pharaoh deserved whatever he got, put yourself in his shoes. His answer was not unreasonable. Slavery was accepted, and slaves were a recognized asset at the time. Everybody had slaves. Authorizing a mass exodus of the slaves in Egypt would have caused a massive write-off, jeopardizing the economy and the willingness of investors to build future pyramids. Slaves, like any asset, are depreciated over what accountants call their "useful life." Let them go before that life is used and you have to write off the remainder immediately. Ask any accountant and he or she will confirm that Pharaoh was in a tough spot here. The only practical answer was "no."

So Pharaoh said no and God hit him with the first salvo. It turned out that Pharaoh was a wimp, and at the first sign of trouble he forgot about the accounting and said, "I give up, go on and get out of here." I'm not making this up. That's what the Bible says, and that is as far as this matter needed to go. God had shown His power, and the Jews were free.

Not so fast. The Egyptians hadn't suffered enough. God hardened Pharaoh's heart and made him change his mind and say no. Pharaoh did what God made him do, and Wham! God hit him with another plague. The poor king tried to give in again, and God again intervened, and made him say no. Wham! God hit him with another punishment. God didn't stop until, as the grand finale, he killed the first-born son in every Egyptian house in the entire country. God also killed the first-born animal in each Egyptian household. The written record does not explain the roles either the children or the animals played in the mistreatment of the slaves, but it must have been pretty bad.

It was a rough night to be an animal. Each Jewish family had to slaughter one of their animals and mark their door jams with its blood so that God would know not to kill any of the children or animals of that household. The written record is unsatisfactory here too and doesn't explain why marking the doors with "ink" or "paint" would not have worked, or if God really needed blood, why families couldn't have shared. You could mark a lot of doors with the blood of a single goat.

This is one tough Supreme Being. He didn't play favorites either. He also was tough on His own. He sent His son down to preach love, and had him nailed to a piece of wood as a lesson to us to love each other. God may have been too optimistic about the ability of the people of that time to understand complex messages. It isn't easy to understand that having His son nailed to a piece of wood meant that we should all love each other. Most people thought He was trying to lead by example. As a result, thousands more were nailed to pieces of wood in the years that followed. Sadly, included among them were many who had tried to teach the new gospel of love.

Now, through the hermit in Central Park, God was directing attention back to Exodus. I thought that this must be a warning of what might happen if we didn't stop fighting with one another. I was no expert at interpretation of divine acts, so I went back to see the hermit.

I asked the hermit if I were correct that God had wanted me to read Exodus as a warning of what would happen if we didn't stop the violence in the Middle East. He nodded. "But how do we create a peace if the religious leaders on both sides speak in God's name against acceptance and compromise?" I asked. "Can't God tell them to stop misquoting Him?"

Again the hermit was sparing with his words. He listened to my question and remained silent for several minutes as if in conversation with someone else. Then he said, "God will offer mankind a second chance. Gather the religious leaders for a walk in the wilderness. God will occupy them for five years. During this time you must find peace."

I protested one last time. "He spent forty years in the wilderness with Moses," I said. "Five years is too short. Why can't we have longer?"

"He liked Moses," the hermit replied. "They used to have long talks. God says he knew Moses and He knows the current leaders, and the current leaders are not Moses! He said you should be thankful that He is willing to spend five years with those assholes."

I couldn't resist. "He really said assholes?" I asked. The hermit stared at me. "You've never talked to Him directly, have you?" he asked. I replied that I had not, and he continued, "When He gets worked up He swears like a sailor. I've been thrown out of all sorts of places for quoting Him too literally. Why do you think I'm a hermit?"

I began spreading the word that God was willing to give Middle East peace a second chance and was inviting all the leading religious leaders to a second "Walk in the Wilderness with God" to discuss the matter. The hermit gave me a box of invitations. They were nicely printed on good parchment. They had been purchased at Bloomingdale's according to the receipt which was still in the bag. In it, the leaders were asked to meet Him on the Sabbath and bring their own staffs. It was signed, simply, "God."

There was a lot of confusion. First, no one could agree on what day the Sabbath fell. The hermit responded to my request for clarification by telling me that God meant Monday, which seemed to throw them all for a loop. A good number of them also misunderstood what God had meant by telling them to bring their staffs and showed up with large entourages. Both they and their staffs were sent packing. True men of religion knew that God meant a large wooden stick when He used the term staff.

Finally, the religious leaders were all assembled and they marched into the desert. Their absence made it possible to talk, but the issues were complex. Each side wanted the same land and was willing to kill for it. No principled rationale to allocate it was ever acceptable to all whose agreement was necessary. We were running out of time, a fact that the hermit reminded me of constantly.

It was blind luck that my daughter interrupted my reflections, complaining that I was ignoring her. She asked that we play the game Monopoly. For those of you unfamiliar with the game, the object is to acquire more land than everyone else, form monopolies, and charge everyone else more rent than they can afford to pay. You win by taking all their money and property, leaving them totally destitute and homeless. The game is not only enjoyable; it is a great teaching tool for our future citizens.

I found myself grinning broadly. Monopoly is a means of allocating property among players that is totally dependent on luck and devoid of any principle. It was exactly what I needed! Why not use the same approach to allocate disputed Middle Eastern land?

I felt hopeful for the first time. Anything that could end the conflict would unleash pent up value so great that each of the parties would receive land more valuable than all of the land would be worth to them under current circumstances. We also could create a Real Estate Investment Trust (REIT), jointly owned by all of the parties, and designed to capitalize on the explosion of property values peace would bring.

The REIT of course would have been fortunate enough to know about the peace deal before it was announced, and it would have acquired as much land as possible shortly beforehand. Citizens in the affected countries would get shares in the REIT and could trade those shares to get villas in Italy, townhouses in San Francisco, apartments in Paris, or—for those who wanted—building lots in the Sinai. Call it grandstanding if you will, but we also would give God shares in the REIT. We make no claim that this would motivate Him to push up share prices, but c'mon, what do you think?

Allocating the land this way would be so free of logic that it could not be said to embrace the views of either side. I am not naïve; there is a lot of emotion tied up in ownership of particular pieces of land. To many, land is not fungible. But if all men are brothers, wouldn't you be prepared to share that land with your brother? What if he said he was sorry for getting you in trouble when you were kids? Besides, what choice do we really have? If you don't want to try this, then come up with something, anything that might work.

During the time of the Pharaohs, God used the weapons of the day to torment the Egyptians. I'm not minimizing the unpleasantness of dealing with rivers of blood and locusts, but He now has access to chemical weapons. This is no time to make Him angry.

Who knows, if both sides laughed at the same things, that could be something to build upon.

I don't dwell on death. I do think about it every once in awhile. In a memoir such as this, published before my death, there are two approaches one can take to cover events such as one's death which have not yet occurred. One can count on a sequel, and therefore do nothing more than try to pique the curiosity of your readers. Alternatively, one can travel through time to the future, taking careful notes on what happens and paying especially close attention to what people say about you at your funeral, and then come back to the present and write faithfully what you find in your notes, even though you don't remember any of it happening. I don't think there will be a sequel to this book, and so of course I took the second path. This is what I found in my notebook.

NINETEENTH INTERLUDE:
PASSWORD TO HEAVEN

Death should not be sad. If we believed that death marks the beginning of an eternal "deathtime" of heavenly delights for those who lived as they should, then it is cause for celebration! We should have a party!

But we don't. We gather at gravesites, delivering eulogies that describe how wonderful the deceased was while expressing grief over his/her death. We extend our deepest sympathy to the family. Greeting cards are a mirror on our culture and confirm that we are sad. It's pointless to argue with Hallmark; they know us better than we know ourselves.

Something is wrong here. Why aren't we looking for cards that read, "Congratulations on the Death of your (fill in the husband, wife, father, mother, etc.)," with joyous lyrics and jokes on the inside? Protest all you want; the fact is that we don't really believe in heaven. Our emotions give us away.

It would be great if heaven were real. I would love to see if I would tire of an eternity of great food, friends, love, sex, chocolate, wine, music, books, massages and pasta. The list is really definitional; if any of these things were missing, then it wouldn't be heaven.

The problem is that there is absolutely nothing to suggest that our idyllic view of an after life is anything more than wishful thinking. Dust to dust is probably more accurate. I hope I'm wrong.

Perhaps it was my hopes that led me to have the dream I had about heaven. It began with my arrival at heaven's gate. I must have died but I didn't remember how. Just as well. Dying is far more frightening than death. Now I was dead and ready to enjoy myself. There were incredible aromas wafting over heaven's outer walls. It was just before lunchtime, and I imagined what it must taste like. I couldn't wait.

There was a Saint somebody or other with a clipboard, and I went over to him and asked how long it was going to be before I could get in? Perhaps he could move things quickly so that I could get some of the lunch?

"I'll be glad to help," he said with a gracious smile. "Come over here and we'll get started."

I walked towards him and found myself standing in front of what looked to be an ATM machine. The name of a Savings and Loan in Texas had been scratched through, and the word "Heaven" had been painted over it in crude letters. The saint spoke again, with a hint of pride in his voice. "Aren't these great? We picked them up for free during the Savings and Loan crisis. They really have improved our admissions practices. Go ahead and enter your personal identification number into the machine."

This seemed odd. This morning, I had forgotten my password at the bank. Or more precisely, I couldn't remember which one of the dozens of passwords I had established for various purposes was the one to be used for the bank. I said in my dream, "Personal identification number?"

"Yes, what you probably think of as your life PIN."

"I don't have one," I said "Wait. That's not right. I have dozens of PINs. But I don't believe I have one for my life."

The saint gave a nervous laugh. "Of course you have one. Everyone has one. They are assigned at birth to the soul of every person. You wouldn't be here if you didn't have one."

"I'm sorry, but I am here, and I don't have one. Or at least I don't remember ever having one, or ever even seeing one," I said. "Where would it have been?"

The saint definitely became agitated. "But this is not possible. How could you lose it? It's given out at birth, at baptism, at last rites and on special occasions in between. We've even started putting it on those tags you find on your mattress that warn you not to remove them."

I dreamt that I answered: "I wasn't baptized. I haven't received last rites. And I always remove the tags from my mattresses. I never saw the password."

The saint took a deep breath and let it out slowly. "I'm very sorry. We made a mistake bringing you here without verifying that you had the proper identification. We have to take you back. You will get a new PIN and a new body. It means living another life."

It was starting to dawn on me that this was really serious. I tried again. "Please. I liked life but I'm ready for heaven."

"Not without a PIN," he said. "This is not something that can be changed. In fact, as of the beginning of the year, knowledge of your

PIN is the primary criterion for entry. It cannot be waived without His personal permission."

This was getting more incredible all the time. "Do you mean to say that remembering a stupid number is the ticket to heaven? Doesn't being good or bad even matter?" I asked.

The saint looked at me as if I were a very slow student. Then, giving a sigh, he explained, "Not to us. It still matters to Santa Claus."

I stared with my mouth open without speaking, which is what I do when I don't know what to say. I don't like how I look when I do that, so I quickly edited my dream, and this time I looked thoughtful yet doubtful. He saw my look, which was a pretty powerful look, and became defensive.

"I forget how cynical you people have become! Of course he exists. I left him not ten minutes ago. Adults become so convinced that he doesn't that they lose the ability to see him. Do you really think that all adults are so smart, and all children so dumb, that the adults could convince the children he exists if he really didn't? I don't think so."

I looked around me to see if this was all a prank, with my wife and friends ready to pounce. None of this made any sense. "Let me try it again," I said. "You're telling me that the only thing relevant to getting into heaven is my knowledge of my PIN number, which I don't have? And that even if I were Mother Theresa, I couldn't get in without it?"

The saint smiled with delight, pleased that I was "getting it." Then he added, "Of course, this oversimplifies it a bit. God does what God wants, but absent His intervention, then yes, you have it right."

"You mentioned Mother Theresa," he continued, "She's a great example. She didn't know what a PIN was and had to go into a new body and come back a second time. It was very strange seeing her as an evangelist, but that was what she was in her next life. Talk about a long shot for entry. But she has a remarkable soul, and she made it back. She is the first and only evangelist that has ever made it to heaven! God says that they talk about hell so much they deserve to see it firsthand."

My mind was awhirl with all the fantastic things I was hearing. I needed to regroup. I had tried to live my life the way my parents had told me I should, and now realized that they had goofed! I should have done memory exercises rather than memorizing my prayers.

The more I thought about it, the angrier I became. "This makes no sense!" I said. "Good people will be turned away, and some undeserving bad people will get in."

"If you can define good and bad, you're ahead of me," he replied. "To many on earth, you are good. Others think you so bad that they want to kill you. Don't talk to me about good and bad unless you are prepared to explain what it means when you say it." He paused, and I thought he looked tired and old. "You make the same arguments we made to Him. The problem was that once you start putting footnotes on the Ten Commandments, all objective measures of 'good' and 'bad' are lost, and the whole thing starts getting very confusing. The commandment says 'thou shalt not kill,' but somehow it became acceptable for some to say killing was the way to please God and get to heaven. Nothing makes Him so angry as watching people violate the Ten Commandments and say that they did it for Him."

He paused again and looked at his watch. "Would you look at the time! I'm sorry, but we must get moving. I'm going to give you your choice," he said, checking his clipboard. "You could be born to a refugee in Afghanistan or to an out-of-work peasant woman with no husband or means of support in Mexico."

I felt sick. "Is that the best you can do?" I asked, not hiding my disappointment.

He gave me a stern look. "These are great choices," he insisted. "With lives like these, you are almost certain to get back to heaven in no time! You're going to be poor, under-nourished and abused by others. Were I to send you back to a comfortable existence in the United States, you would have all sorts of chances to go astray. Here, for a short lifetime of squalor, you will be on the fast track to eternal bliss."

I had one nagging concern. "What if I forget my personal identification number again?" I asked. "It seems like I will just keep going around and around in circles."

The saint gave it some thought. "I think Mexico is the right place for you. When it comes to freeing souls from the bodies of their poorest citizens, there are few places that can match it. It's also heavily Catholic, and we are going to be including a reminder of the PIN number as a part of the last rites."

As we started to walk, his cell phone rang. He listened, and then grabbed my arm and said, "Come, there is no time to lose. We must get you ready to be launched into a new body."

"What's the rush?" I asked.

"You are scheduled to join your new body, so to speak, at the moment of conception. That's to make certain no other soul grabs that body first. But as you can imagine, the timing of conception can be very unpredictable. That is why we rarely use it. It requires us to watch the man and woman carefully and deliver the soul at exactly the right time. Your parents-to-be are on a first date, and we thought that we had more time. But your mother is very innocent and your father is handsome and very persistent."

He paused. "She's a beautiful lady, your mother." He paused again, and then almost yelled, "This is it! He's in! Man he is fast!" A few moments later the saint muttered, "Really fast." A green light turned on and a door swung open. I imagined that the room we were in looked very similar to the interior of a plane used for skydiving. He turned to me, gave me a quick hug, and said, "See you soon." I jumped out the open door and was gone.

I am a young Mexican boy. I don't know why they asked me to write something in this book. Maybe it is because I have been very sick recently and the doctors don't expect me to live. It's not really a surprise. My father and mother didn't marry, and he didn't stick around. That's a big thing here, and she was told to leave her parents' home by her father when I was born. Now we live in a garbage dump with others who don't have a home. It's okay except when my mother goes to town to try to find work and the bigger boys around here steal the lunch she leaves for me. I can't tell her that because she would worry too much. For now I eat garbage. It's not as bad as it sounds. I've learned to spot garbage from the rich homes. There's always something that's pretty good. But you have to be careful not to eat anything too old. I must have eaten something bad last week because my stomach has never hurt so much.

I think things will get better. I have a plan. I've almost finished building my knife from a piece of metal I found. When it is sharp enough I plan to surprise the bullies who take my lunch. If I kill one, the others will run, because they're cowards when they don't have you outnumbered. Once I start eating real food I'll get stronger and will be able to get a job. Then when we have enough money we'll get a real home.

The boy died two days later, killed with a makeshift knife during a fight over food with an older, much larger boy. There was no investigation into the death because it didn't seem to matter to anyone but his grieving mother, and she didn't seem to care why he had died, but only that he had. The world noticed neither his life nor his death. I became so angry that I woke myself up.

As I lay in bed, eyes closed, I was utterly convinced I had been the boy and had just died in Mexico. I was disabused when, still groggy, I got up and took a few steps on the Mexican tile floor in our sitting room and banged my toe hard against the molding around the bathroom door. I howled and grabbed my foot and felt alive!

My wife called out to see if I was okay, and not getting an immediate answer, turned on a light. I looked at her. Perhaps it was the lingering effect of my dream, but she looked uncommonly beautiful to me just then. Making love was an infrequent event between us, but that morning we made a great start at making up for lost time. Afterwards, she put on a robe and said she would go down and make me breakfast. I told her I would take a quick shower. I stepped into the stall and began humming. I felt alive and happy. She came back upstairs when I got out of the shower and looked at me with a questioning expression.

"Are you okay?" she asked.

"Never better," I responded. I told her that I had woken up thinking that I had died as a poor Mexican boy. "It was so real that I can't believe it didn't happen." My wife just looked at me, waiting for me to continue. "And that means that we need to contribute more to charity, not just our money but our time. And we ought to take a vacation, and make love and enjoy our lives like we have never done."

She looked even more puzzled. "Listen," I said, "there's a lot I need to tell you. I'm going to call the office and tell them I won't be in today. Let's go out and have something to eat. Didn't you say that there was a wonderful little Mexican restaurant that just opened down in the village?"

On the way to the restaurant we talked about my dream. It was hard to describe my dream without sounding silly. But she accepted it because it was so strange. She also made me feel much better by telling me for the first time that she had a dream that kept repeating itself, which made me feel more normal. In her dream, she came back as a cockroach living under Herman Munster's refrigerator. I'm glad I don't understand what it means. "Stay away from vacuums," I said.

We agreed to hedge our bets and buy a new mattress, with tags, and to do much, much more to help people who needed help. I'm not being preachy, but my experience, or dream, about the young boy had made this important to me. It felt like a new beginning. Lighthearted and more optimistic than I had been in a long time, I took my wife's hand and pulled her closer. When she was within reach, I put my arms around her and we kissed. After all, there was no requirement that one wait until one dies to experience heaven.

We kissed long enough for people to stare at us. I didn't care. Then, we entered the restaurant, surrounded by aromas of food being expertly prepared that were delightful and surprisingly familiar at the same time.

An old, bad joke tries to create mirth out of two things totally lacking in humor: (1) the propensity of German writers, especially German philosophers, to use very long sentences, and (2) German grammar, which places verbs at the end of those sentences. The joke is that a critic who has just read the first two volumes of a three-volume book on German philosophy is asked what he thinks of it thus far. He replies that he doesn't yet know what to think because all the verbs are in the third volume.

As I promised, it's not that funny. For whatever reason, I remember that joke while forgetting ones far better. One night when I could neither sleep nor write, I began thinking about German grammar and wondering why the creators of this language decided to place the verbs at the end of sentences.

My first hypothesis was that this had been a tactical decision influenced by the German military during one of the country's aggressive periods. While their neighbors listened to the German diplomats, waiting patiently for them to reveal the verbs so that they could learn what the Germans were doing, going to do, or had done, the German Army would slip across the border, announce the annexation of the country and that would be that. Poland normally could be taken in a single sentence, although to be fair, only if that sentence had been written by Hegel.

A better explanation of the placement of German verbs is that the Germans simply in different ways their thoughts have come to think. (That sentence was for the benefit of my German readers. I saw one of them smile when he read it and heard him whisper to his friend, "Now that was the first sentence that any sense made.")

While this epilogue may not seem to be going anywhere, we have in fact covered the ground necessary for me to explain why, emulating German grammar, I waited for the end of the book to explain what I hope you will take from it. I wrote what I wrote without a real purpose other than to lift my own spirits. Only when I laid it out end to end did I realize that there seemed to be a point to all this worth sharing.

Writing this book was my entertainment during a difficult passage in my life. Most of the stories, including the silly ones intended to do nothing more than make you laugh, were written late at night when I had already exhausted the amount of medicine I could safely take that day. I was suffering the full effect of my Parkinson's, which at my stage of progression meant significant muscular rigidity and pain. To make matters worse, I also was paying the price of the medicine's side effects from all the pills I had taken to control the disease earlier in the day. In other words, I was shaking and aching at the same time.

Some of what I wrote was about illness. My early successes in having things published were on that topic. But most of what I wrote, and certainly the part that was more enjoyable for me to write, was about having fun. Like the character in Jack London's book *The Star Rover* who used his mind to escape his shackles, writing became to me a means of escape into a world where I could move and laugh without restriction. I did more than survive in this private world; I learned to have fun.

It struck me odd that people called me brave for trying to enjoy my life, as if the "normal" thing to have done would have been to curl up in a ball and let the world know how much I was suffering. I confess to enjoying myself more now, even knowing that I have a troublesome disease, than I did when I was a successful lawyer who "had it all," oblivious to the health issues about to rear their ugly little heads.

Illness causes a marvelous re-ordering of priorities that I badly needed. I had caught the successes I had been chasing and still felt empty. I can't quite reach a point where I can say that I'm glad I have Parkinson's Disease, but I also know that it has had a wonderful as well as a miserable impact on my life. It is troubling to consider what I might have missed if I had continued plodding along, chasing things that gave me little happiness. One can go through life without enjoying it. I learned through illness the importance of enjoying every minute, and sometimes I believe that for all my medical "issues," I get more fun out of the things I am able to do than many without physical handicaps who do more and enjoy themselves less.

I don't question that there are things so horrible (like being eaten by a crocodile) that they cannot be made pleasurable by having a good attitude. But we put much more of life's experiences into this "crocodile" category than is necessary.

Not everyone can count on illness being a wake-up call. The healthy among us are traveling through life without an alarm clock and are in danger of not waking at all. I intend this book to be your alarm clock. Hopefully, by sharing my experiences with you as I have, you will find in these words the same reasons to live life more intensely, without Death breathing down your neck.

I wrote in the interlude "Love" that our bodies reward things good for us with pleasure and bad for us with pain, an evolutionary carrot-and-stick compass to help us survive. Smiling at life, and finding a way to see the humor in everything including one's misadventures, makes one feel, well, wonderful. Giving and receiving real love creates not just pleasure but euphoria as well; being eaten by crocodiles, I suspect, puts any pain I've suffered to shame. People generally remember to stay away from crocodiles without books reminding them. Yet they forget that living life without the joy of a good laugh, or the euphoria of shared love, is the equivalent of staying in the swamp, where it is just a question of time before you become the crocodile's next meal.

Live life for all it's worth, laugh and love, and stay away from crocodiles. As philosophies of life go, you could do worse.

Printed in the United States
75103LV00005B/4-105

9 781934 160008